Diabetes

A practical guide to managing your health

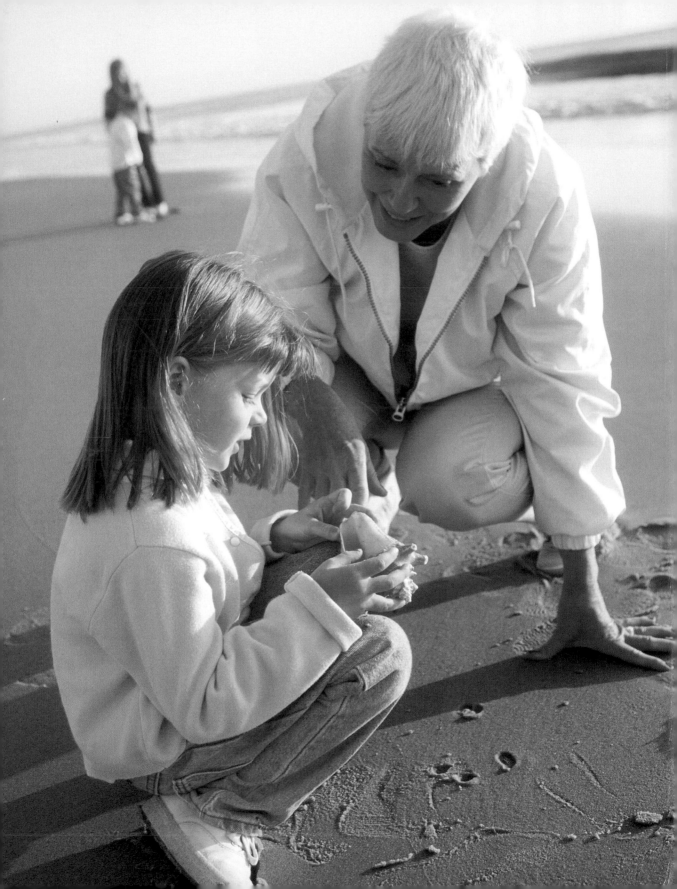

Diabetes

A practical guide to managing your health

Rosemary Walker & Jill Rodgers

London, New York, Munich, Melbourne, Delhi

DORLING KINDERSLEY

Senior Editors Dawn Henderson, Kesta Desmond
Senior Art Editor Catherine MacKenzie
Senior Managing Editor Martyn Page
Managing Art Editor Marianne Markham
DTP Designer Julian Dams
Production Controllers Wendy Penn, Kirsti Rippon
Production Manager Sarah Coltman
Category Publishers Mary Thompson, Corinne Roberts
Art Director Bryn Walls

Produced for Dorling Kindersley by
COOLING BROWN
9–11 High Street, Hampton,
Middlesex TW12 2SA

Managing Editor Amanda Lebentz
Art Editor Tish Jones
Creative Director Arthur Brown

First published in the United Kingdom in 2004
This edition first published 2010 by
Dorling Kindersley Limited, 80 Strand, London WC2R 0RL
A Penguin Company

2 4 6 8 10 9 7 5 3 1

002 - LD014 - September/2010

Every effort has been made to ensure that the information in this book is accurate. The information in this book may not be applicable in each individual case so you are therefore advised to obtain expert medical advice for specific information on personal health matters. Never disregard expert medical advice or delay in receiving advice or treatment due to information obtained from this book. The naming of any product, treatment, or organization in this book does not imply endorsement by the authors, imprimatur, or publisher, nor does the omission of such names indicate disapproval. The publisher, authors, and imprimatur cannot accept legal responsibility for any personal injury or other damage or loss arising from any use or misuse of the information and advice in this book.

A CIP catalogue record for this book is available from the British Library.

ISBN 978-1-4053-4428-9

Reproduced by Colourscan, Singapore
Printed in China

Discover more at
www.dk.com

Foreword

Having diabetes has an impact on every aspect of a person's life. Our aim in writing this book has been to provide useful, practical information to help people living with diabetes to make decisions that enable them to live successfully with the condition. Diabetes cannot be taken lightly, but there are ways of managing it so that it doesn't interfere with hopes, dreams, and aspirations for work and play. We hope that we have presented the most valuable and effective ways of managing the condition in the following pages.

In our experience, people learn a great deal about day-to-day life with diabetes from other people with the condition. Because of this, we have included people's real experiences, thoughts, and feelings throughout this book. We hope that those we have chosen to illustrate key aspects of living with diabetes will ring true for readers and be of benefit to them. Collecting these experiences has taught us much along the way, and we are especially grateful to the people who shared their stories so willingly and honestly.

We are aware that diabetes conjures up different thoughts and emotions in everyone and that each person's journey with diabetes is an individual experience. However, as we were collecting the stories of people's lives with diabetes, one quote summed up how it is possible to incorporate looking after diabetes into everyday life and continue to adapt to what is an ever-changing condition:

'To seek, to strive, to find, and not to yield.'

Rosemary Walker

Rosemary Walker

Jill Rodgers

Jill Rodgers

Contents

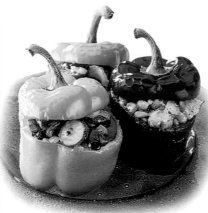

WHAT IS DIABETES?

Understanding diabetes 10
What is diabetes? 10
Types of diabetes 12
Why does diabetes
  develop? 16

Symptoms and diagnosis 18
Recognizing diabetes 18
Diagnosing diabetes 21

Looking after your diabetes 22
Monitoring
  blood glucose 22
Controlling
  blood glucose 23
Working with your health
  professional 26
Long-term complications 26

FOOD, DRINK, AND PHYSICAL ACTIVITY

Healthy eating and drinking 30
Healthy eating principles 30
Food groups 33
Vitamins and minerals 37
Fibre 38
Diabetic products and
  sweeteners 38

Drinks 38
Healthier cooking 40
Eating out 41

Weight and diabetes 44
Why weight matters 44
How to lose weight 47

Physical activity 52
Being more active 52
Managing physical activity
  and diabetes 56

CONTROLLING YOUR BLOOD GLUCOSE

Monitoring blood glucose 62
Understanding blood
  glucose levels 62
Monitoring equipment 67
Performing a blood
  glucose test 70
Responding to test results 74

Tablets and other medication 76
Controlling diabetes
  with medication 76
Types of medication 78

Insulin 82
Controlling diabetes
  with insulin 82
Types of insulin 84
Insulin regimens 87
Adjusting doses
  of insulin 90
Insulin equipment 95
Choosing your injection
  site 97
How to inject yourself 98
Insulin and equipment
  care 99
Advances in treatment 100

Hypoglycaemia 102
What is hypoglycaemia? 102
Causes and
  prevention 102
Symptoms 105
Treatment 106
The recovery period 108

Hyperglycaemia 110
What is hyperglycaemia? 110
Causes and
  prevention 110
Symptoms 112
Treatment 112
Risks 113

LIVING WITH DIABETES

Day-to-day life 116

Staying motivated 116
Work 118
Driving 120
Holidays and travel 122
Sex and
  relationships 126

Looking after yourself 128

Footcare 128
When you become ill 130
Long-term drug
  treatments 133
Going into hospital 134

Women's health 136

Female hormones 136
Cystitis and thrush 137
Pregnancy 138
Giving birth 142
Gestational
  diabetes 144
Life with a new baby 146

Benefiting from health care 148

Keeping yourself
  informed 148
Getting the
  most from your
  appointments 149

CHILDREN AND TEENAGERS

Babies and young children 154

Diabetes, your child, and you 154
Eating and drinking 156
Blood glucose control 157
Coping with illness 161

School-age children 162

Diabetes, your child, and you 162
Eating and drinking 164
Blood glucose control 167
Life at school 169

Teenagers and young adults 170

Diabetes, your teenager,
  and you 170
Your feelings as a teenager 173
Eating and drinking 176
Blood glucose control 176
Getting on with your life 178
Talking to other people 182

POSSIBLE LONG-TERM COMPLICATIONS

Depression 186

Understanding depression 186

Eye conditions 190

Retinopathy 190
Cataracts 194
Living with reduced vision 195

Kidney conditions 196

Nephropathy 196

Foot conditions 200

Peripheral neuropathy 200
Peripheral ischaemia 202

Cardiovascular conditions 206

High blood pressure 206
Hyperlipidaemia 208
Coronary heart disease 209
Stroke 210
Peripheral vascular disease 211

Other conditions 212

Lipohypertrophy 212
Erectile dysfunction 213
Autonomic neuropathy 215

Glossary 216

Useful addresses 218
Index 219
Acknowledgments 224

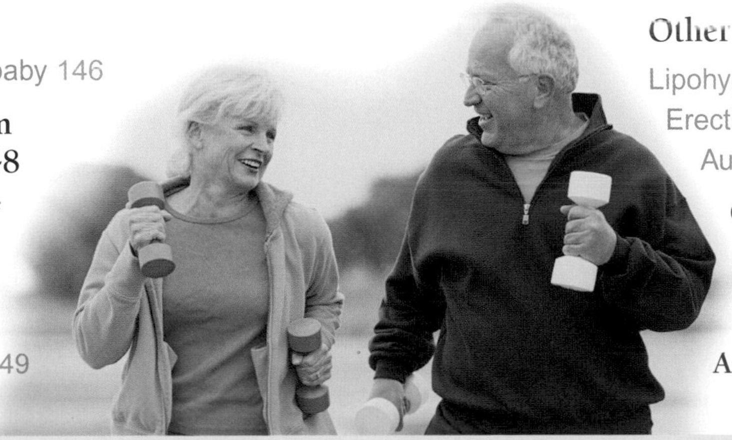

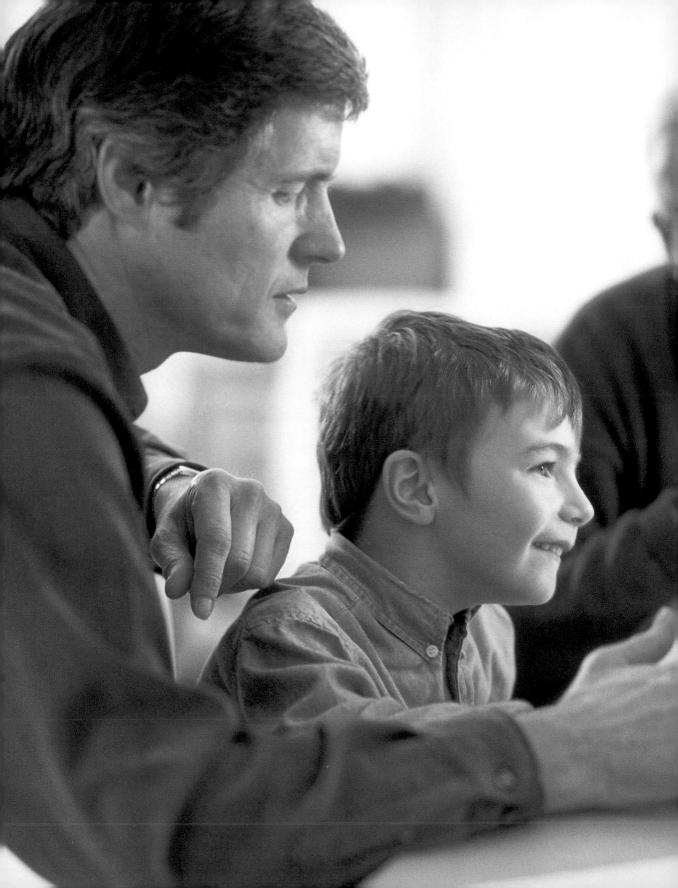

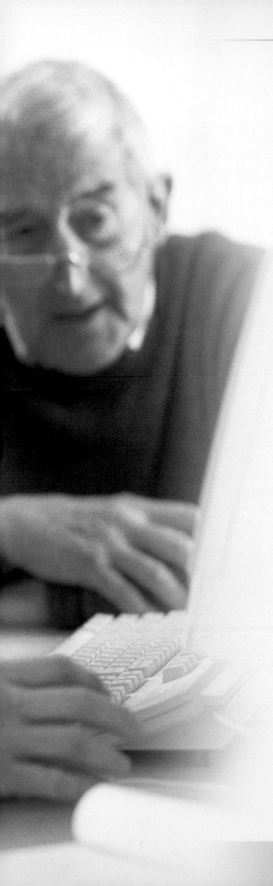

What is diabetes?

Today about 200 million people worldwide have diabetes, and this number is increasing by more than 20 million each year.

If you or someone close to you has diabetes, it's important to understand as much as you can about the condition. This chapter gives an overview of diabetes, explaining how the healthy body uses glucose (sugar) and how a person with diabetes is unable to use glucose in this way.

There is no single cause of diabetes but there are risk factors that, in combination, increase your chances of developing the condition. These risk factors can be related to your genes, the environment, or your lifestyle. How quickly you are diagnosed with diabetes depends, in part, on the nature and severity of your symptoms.

Although diabetes has an impact on your day-to-day health, it can also have serious effects on your long-term health. If your blood glucose level is regularly raised over a period of years, this can cause damage to your eyes, kidneys, feet, and heart, for example. This is why effective long-term management of your diabetes is so important.

Understanding diabetes

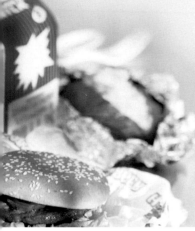

Understanding diabetes means knowing how the hormone insulin usually controls your blood glucose level and what happens inside your body when this control breaks down. There are different types of diabetes, but in each type glucose accumulates in your blood to a level that could be harmful to your health. Whether you develop diabetes, and which type you develop, is the result of a combination of inherited and environmental factors.

Myth OR TRUTH?

MYTH
Eating too much sugar can cause diabetes.

TRUTH
Diabetes is caused by a combination of inherited and environmental factors. Sugar itself doesn't cause diabetes but it can make you put on weight. Being overweight increases your risk of developing Type 2 diabetes. So keeping your weight healthy for your height can help to prevent Type 2 diabetes.

What is diabetes?

Diabetes is a condition in which your body cannot control the level of glucose (sugar) in your blood because your pancreas does not produce insulin, does not produce enough insulin, or your body cells are resistant to the action of insulin. Therefore, when your blood glucose level rises, the glucose cannot get into your body cells and so they are deprived of their usual source of energy. Your body responds by trying to eliminate excess glucose from your blood and by using fat and protein (from muscle) as alternative sources of energy. This disrupts your bodily processes and can cause some of the symptoms of diabetes (see pp.18–19).

How the healthy body uses glucose

When you eat carbohydrate foods such as bread, rice, potatoes, cereals or sugar, they are broken down into glucose during digestion. Glucose moves from the intestines into the bloodstream and then enters the body's cells where it is burned as fuel – it powers your entire body, from the muscles to the brain, and is the body's primary source of energy. Glucose is also stored in the liver and muscles in the form of glycogen.

Two of the main hormones that control blood glucose are insulin and glucagon. Both are produced in the pancreas, a gland that lies behind the stomach. There are clusters of cells in the pancreas called the islets of Langerhans; within these are two types of hormone-producing cells, alpha and beta cells: alpha cells produce glucagon; beta cells produce insulin.

There is a constant background level of insulin in your body but when your blood glucose level rises – after eating, for example – extra insulin is released by your beta cells. Insulin acts like a key, unlocking

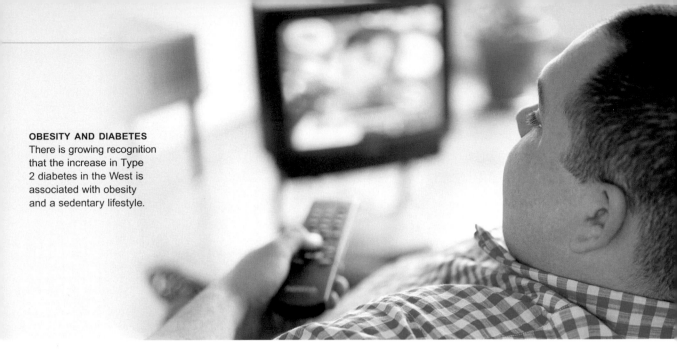

OBESITY AND DIABETES
There is growing recognition that the increase in Type 2 diabetes in the West is associated with obesity and a sedentary lifestyle.

body cells so that glucose can enter. When your blood glucose level falls – after a period without food, for example – your alpha cells release more glucagon, which converts glycogen in your liver back to glucose. This enters your bloodstream and your blood glucose level rises again. Insulin and glucagon work together constantly in this way to ensure that your blood glucose level stays within a close range of 4–6 millimoles of glucose per litre of blood. As a result, whether you have eaten a lot of carbohydrate or a little, your body has the constant supply of energy it needs to work properly.

What goes wrong in diabetes?

When you have diabetes, the finely tuned system that regulates blood glucose fails because you don't produce insulin, or you don't produce enough of it, or your body is resistant

THE HEALTHY BODY'S RESPONSE TO GLUCOSE

Glucose is the body's primary energy source. The quantity of glucose in your blood is carefully regulated by two pancreatic hormones, insulin and glucagon. This means that, despite variations in the amount of carbohydrate you eat, your body has a constant supply of glucose from which to produce energy.

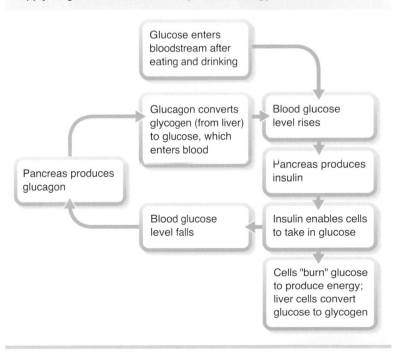

Glucose enters bloodstream after eating and drinking

Blood glucose level rises

Pancreas produces insulin

Glucagon converts glycogen (from liver) to glucose, which enters blood

Pancreas produces glucagon

Insulin enables cells to take in glucose

Blood glucose level falls

Cells "burn" glucose to produce energy; liver cells convert glucose to glycogen

to insulin. As a result, glucose cannot pass into your cells to be burned for energy, so it builds up in the blood. This leads to an abnormally high blood glucose level.

A high blood glucose level

When you have a raised blood glucose level you may experience symptoms such as passing large amounts of urine and excessive thirst. This is because your body removes excess glucose by filtering it through your kidneys and into your urine (the thirst is a result of dehydration). Also, because your body cannot use glucose properly for energy, it obtains energy by breaking down your muscle and fat stores. This can cause weight loss and, in the case of rapid fat breakdown, toxic chemicals building up in your blood. Unfortunately, a raised blood glucose level does not always produce symptoms, and only a blood glucose test (see pp.70–73) can tell you that it is high. A blood glucose level that is consistently high over a period of years can damage the body's tissues, leading to complications involving your eyes, kidneys, feet, heart, blood vessels, and nerves.

Types of diabetes

There are two main types of diabetes: Type 1 and Type 2, the latter being the most common. Although they are both types of diabetes, Type 1 and Type 2 are very different conditions. There are also other types of diabetes that affect a minority of people: Maturity Onset Diabetes of the Young (MODY), gestational diabetes, and rarer forms that are related to infections, medications, and pancreas disease or damage.

Type 1 diabetes

Previously known as "juvenile onset" or "insulin-dependent" diabetes, Type 1 diabetes affects fewer than 1 in 5 people with diabetes. It usually appears during childhood, teenage years, or early adulthood. If you have Type 1 diabetes, you don't produce any insulin because the beta cells in

THE PANCREAS
Lying deep within the abdomen and behind the stomach, the pancreas is a gland that secretes all of the body's insulin – one of the hormones that regulates the level of glucose in the blood. The cells in the pancreas that manufacture and release insulin are called beta cells and are found in the islets of Langerhans.

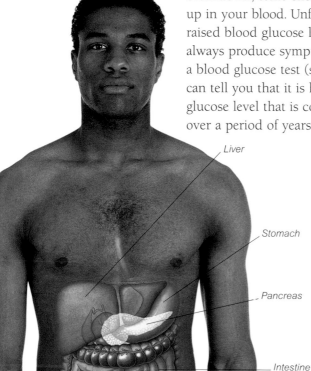

Liver

Stomach

Pancreas

Intestine

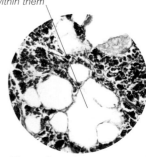

Islets of Langerhans

White spaces show the breakdown of the islets of Langerhans and destruction of beta cells within them

Tissue from a healthy pancreas

Tissue from the pancreas of a person with Type 1 diabetes

TYPE 1 DIABETES – YOUR BODY'S RESPONSE TO GLUCOSE

If you have Type 1 diabetes, your pancreas does not produce any insulin. This means that your blood glucose level rises unchecked and your body is deprived of its primary energy source. This results in fatigue, lack of energy, passing large amounts of urine, dehydration, thirst, and weight loss. To compensate for the lack of glucose, your body breaks down fat and protein (from muscle) as an alternative energy source. This can lead to a potentially life-threatening condition called diabetic ketoacidosis. Your pancreas still produces glucagon, another pancreatic hormone involved in blood glucose control.

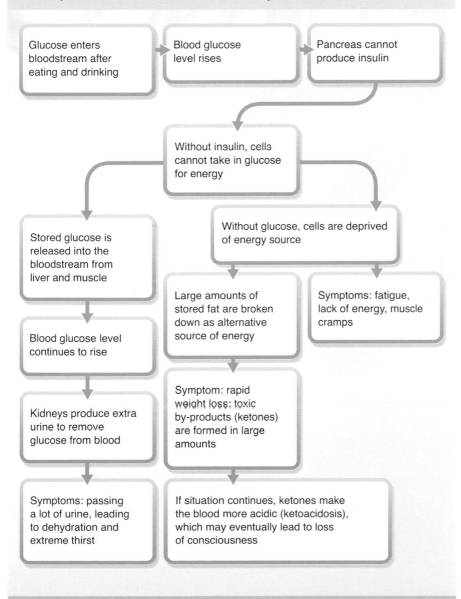

Glucose enters bloodstream after eating and drinking

Blood glucose level rises

Pancreas cannot produce insulin

Without insulin, cells cannot take in glucose for energy

Stored glucose is released into the bloodstream from liver and muscle

Without glucose, cells are deprived of energy source

Large amounts of stored fat are broken down as alternative source of energy

Symptoms: fatigue, lack of energy, muscle cramps

Blood glucose level continues to rise

Kidneys produce extra urine to remove glucose from blood

Symptom: rapid weight loss; toxic by-products (ketones) are formed in large amounts

Symptoms: passing a lot of urine, leading to dehydration and extreme thirst

If situation continues, ketones make the blood more acidic (ketoacidosis), which may eventually lead to loss of consciousness

If you have Type 1 diabetes, you don't produce any insulin because the beta cells in your pancreas have been destroyed.

Myth OR
TRUTH?

MYTH

Type 2 diabetes is less serious than Type 1.

TRUTH

In some ways, Type 2 diabetes is more serious because people may have it for years before being diagnosed. This means that they may already have developed long-term complications without being aware of them.

The rising incidence of obesity that is associated with a sedentary Western lifestyle may trigger Type 2 diabetes.

TYPE 2 DIABETES – YOUR BODY'S RESPONSE TO GLUCOSE

If you have Type 2 diabetes, your body cells are resistant to the action of insulin and/or your pancreas produces decreasing amounts of insulin. As a result, your blood glucose level becomes progressively higher over time and your body cells receive an inadequate supply of glucose – your body's primary energy source. This may result in a range of symptoms including fatigue, lack of energy, passing large amounts of urine, thirst, and gradual weight loss. To make up for insufficient glucose, your body may break down fat and protein (from muscle) as additional energy sources. Because your pancreas still produces some insulin, however, your body doesn't become entirely dependent on fat as an energy source (as in Type 1 diabetes) and you do not develop diabetic ketoacidosis.

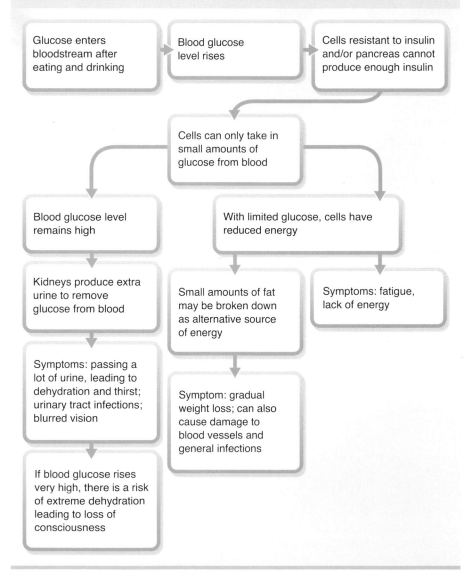

Glucose enters bloodstream after eating and drinking

Blood glucose level rises

Cells resistant to insulin and/or pancreas cannot produce enough insulin

Cells can only take in small amounts of glucose from blood

Blood glucose level remains high

With limited glucose, cells have reduced energy

Kidneys produce extra urine to remove glucose from blood

Small amounts of fat may be broken down as alternative source of energy

Symptoms: fatigue, lack of energy

Symptoms: passing a lot of urine, leading to dehydration and thirst; urinary tract infections; blurred vision

Symptom: gradual weight loss; can also cause damage to blood vessels and general infections

If blood glucose rises very high, there is a risk of extreme dehydration leading to loss of consciousness

your pancreas have been destroyed. In most cases, this is the result of an autoimmune response in which your immune system mistakenly treats your beta cells as foreign bodies and attacks them. This response may be triggered by a viral infection. Although Type 1 diabetes seems to develop suddenly, the destruction of beta cells can start months or years earlier. It is not until your beta cells are functioning at less than 10 per cent of their capacity that diabetes symptoms appear.

Type 1 diabetes is treated with insulin, given by injection or via a pump (see pp.82–101). You cannot take insulin in tablet form because it would be destroyed during digestion.

Type 2 diabetes

Previously known as "maturity onset" or "non-insulin-dependent" diabetes, Type 2 diabetes affects 4 in 5 people with diabetes and tends to develop after the age of 40. The rising incidence of obesity that is associated with a sedentary Western lifestyle may trigger Type 2 diabetes. It is also becoming increasingly common for children and teenagers to develop Type 2 diabetes for this reason.

If you have Type 2 diabetes, you produce insulin, but in insufficient amounts and/or your body cells are resistant to the action of insulin. Initially, your pancreas responds to insulin resistance by producing more insulin, but, over time, your pancreas cannot keep up with your body's demand for insulin – this is why the treatment of Type 2 diabetes changes over time. At first, losing weight, healthier eating, and physical activity may keep your blood glucose level well controlled, sometimes for years. When necessary, you are prescribed tablets that increase the amount of insulin in your blood, improve your insulin's function, or change the rate at which carbohydrate is broken down during digestion. Eventually, you are likely to need insulin injections, too.

COMPARING TYPE 1 AND TYPE 2 DIABETES

Although they share some of the same symptoms, Type 1 and Type 2 diabetes are really separate conditions, and there are separate causes and treatments for each.

TYPE 1 DIABETES	TYPE 2 DIABETES
Usually starts in childhood or early adulthood; rarely develops after age 40.	Usually starts in adulthood, often after age 40 but increasingly common at a younger age.
The body doesn't produce insulin because the insulin-producing beta cells in the pancreas have been destroyed.	The body produces insulin but it is resistant to its action. Over time, insulin production progressively declines.
People affected are usually underweight or normal weight.	People affected are usually overweight.
People affected need insulin treatment, as well as care with eating and physical activity.	People affected need care with healthy eating, physical activity, and tablet and insulin treatment.
Passing large amounts of urine, excessive thirst, weight loss, and fatigue can come on quickly and be severe.	Passing large amounts of urine, excessive thirst, weight loss, fatigue, and blurred vision may be gradual, mild or absent.
Diagnosis is usually rapid – within days or weeks of symptoms developing.	Diabetes may not be diagnosed for several years.
Children of people with Type 1 diabetes have a 1–6 per cent chance of developing Type 1 diabetes.	Children of people with Type 2 diabetes have a 14 per cent chance of developing Type 2 diabetes.
Cannot be prevented.	Risk reduced by weight control and regular physical activity.

Maturity Onset Diabetes of the Young (MODY)

This is a rare type of diabetes that affects about 1 in 100 people with diabetes. MODY usually becomes apparent in the teens or 20s. It is similar to Type 2 diabetes but develops only in people with specific genes that cause a defect in the way the insulin-producing cells in the pancreas work. This leads to underproduction of insulin. MODY can be confirmed by genetic testing. Treatment – as with Type 2 diabetes – usually focuses on healthy eating and physical activity first, then tablet treatment and/or insulin if necessary.

Gestational diabetes

This type of diabetes may develop around the 28th week (sixth month) of pregnancy and is the only temporary form of diabetes. For more about gestational diabetes, see pp.144–145.

Why does diabetes develop?

Diabetes has no single cause, but may be caused by a combination of any of the following inherited and environmental factors.

GESTATIONAL DIABETES
The hormonal changes of pregnancy can lead to insulin resistance and temporary diabetes in some women. Gestational diabetes usually disappears when pregnancy is over but can reappear in future pregnancies and greatly increases a woman's risk of developing Type 2 diabetes in later life.

■ **GENES** If you have the specific genes for Type 1 diabetes, you may develop it at some point in your life, although this is not inevitable. If you don't have the genes for Type 1 diabetes, you will not develop it (unless you have your pancreas removed). In Type 2 diabetes there is no specific genetic pattern, but your chances of developing it increase if members of your family have the condition (see opposite). There are also certain genetic syndromes which, although rare, can increase your risk of developing diabetes, the most common being Down's syndrome, which can lead to Type 2 diabetes.

■ **WEIGHT** If you are overweight, you have an increased risk of developing Type 2 diabetes because your body cells may become resistant to insulin. Obesity, defined as weighing 20 per cent more than your ideal body weight (see p.46), further increases your risk. Being overweight does not increase your risk of Type 1 diabetes.

■ **BODY SHAPE** If you carry excess weight around your waist, you have a higher risk of developing Type 2 diabetes (but not Type 1 diabetes) than if you carry excess weight on your hips and thighs (see p.45).

■ **ETHNIC BACKGROUND** If you are of South Asian, African, or Caribbean descent you have five times more chance of developing Type 2 diabetes than people of Caucasian origin (but you are no more likely to develop Type 1 diabetes).

■ **PREGNANCY** When you are pregnant your body increases its blood glucose level in order to cope with the demands of a growing baby, and more insulin is needed. If your body can't produce enough insulin, your blood glucose level remains high and gestational diabetes is diagnosed.

■ **MEDICATIONS** Some medicines can raise your blood glucose level or prevent insulin from working properly. If you take any of these medicines, you have a higher chance of developing Type 2 diabetes.

● Steroids, such as prednisolone and dexamethasone, which are used to treat inflammatory conditions.

● Thiazide diuretics, such as bendroflumethiazide, which are used to remove excess fluid from the body.

● Beta-blockers, such as propranolol, or vasodilators, such as diazoxide, which are used to treat high blood pressure.

● Immunosuppressants, such as ciclosporin, which are used to prevent rejection of organs, following a transplant.

■ **VIRAL INFECTIONS** Specific infections, which may have occurred up to two years earlier, may trigger Type 1 diabetes if you are genetically predisposed to it. A virus can set off an abnormal reaction in which your immune system destroys the insulin-producing cells in your pancreas. Viral infections do not trigger Type 2 diabetes.

■ **DAMAGE TO THE PANCREAS** The following conditions may lead to the development of diabetes.

● Pancreatitis (an inflammation of the pancreas).

● Cystic fibrosis (a genetic condition

CHANCES OF INHERITING DIABETES

Having diabetes in your family increases the risk of you developing it too. This table shows your increased risk of developing diabetes, depending on which of your close relatives has diabetes.

FAMILY MEMBER	YOUR INCREASED RISK
Mother with Type 1	1–2%
Mother with Type 2	14%
Father with Type 1	3–6%
Father with Type 2	14%
Both parents with Type 1	30%
Both parents with Type 2	75%
Sibling with Type 1	6%
Sibling with Type 2	15–25%
Identical twin with Type 1	30%
Identical twin with Type 2	50–100%
No relatives with diabetes	No increased risk

that causes body secretions to be abnormally thick).

● Haemochromatosis (a build-up of excess iron that gradually damages the insulin-producing cells).

● Removal of the pancreas. If your pancreas is removed due to disease, such as cancer, or an accident, Type 1 diabetes develops because you can no longer produce insulin.

■ **HORMONAL DISORDERS** If your body overproduces hormones that oppose the action of insulin, your risk of developing Type 2 diabetes increases. The main hormonal disorders linked with diabetes are Cushing's disease, in which the adrenal glands produce excess steroid hormones, and acromegaly, in which the pituitary gland overproduces growth hormone.

If you carry excess weight around your waist, you have a higher risk of developing Type 2 diabetes.

Symptoms and diagnosis

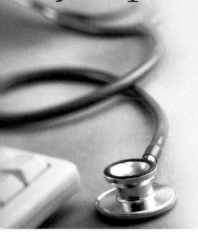

The symptoms of both types of diabetes are similar, but they tend to be more acute at diagnosis in Type 1, and develop more gradually – even over many years – in Type 2. If you think you may have diabetes, see your doctor as soon as possible. The condition is diagnosed with one or more blood tests. If these tests confirm you have diabetes, you will have other tests to assess your health and check for any signs of the long-term complications of diabetes.

Recognizing diabetes

It is more common to notice the symptoms of a high blood glucose level if you have Type 1 diabetes, as the absence of insulin has a dramatic effect on your body. If you have Type 2 diabetes, you still produce some insulin, so your symptoms may be less severe – you may even attribute them to growing older. For example, you may think it's normal to feel tired, or to get up at night to pass urine. Occasionally with Type 2, there are no symptoms at all and diabetes may not even be suspected until you have a routine medical or eye test that reveals early signs of long-term complications. The following are all symptoms of diabetes.

■ **PASSING LARGE AMOUNTS OF URINE FREQUENTLY** When your blood glucose level reaches a certain level, your kidneys filter excess glucose out of your blood. To expel it from your body, more urine is produced, which means that you need to urinate more often. You may not notice this during the day, but you may wake up two or three times a night to pass urine.

■ **DRY MOUTH, EXCESSIVE THIRST** Because you are passing lots of urine you become dehydrated, which causes thirst and a dry mouth. Quenching your thirst with sugary drinks can aggravate the problem by raising your blood glucose even higher, so drink sugar-free drinks.

■ **LACK OF ENERGY** You may feel tired all the time, find it difficult to carry out

My experience

"I couldn't stop passing urine and I had this incredible thirst. One day I was so thirsty that I found myself drinking from the cold water tap while I sat on the toilet." JULIE

COMMENT Passing large amounts of urine frequently and intense thirst are two symptoms of diabetes. When blood glucose reaches 10 millimoles per litre, excess glucose is passed out in the urine. Large amounts of water (to dilute the glucose) are lost, causing dehydration and thirst.

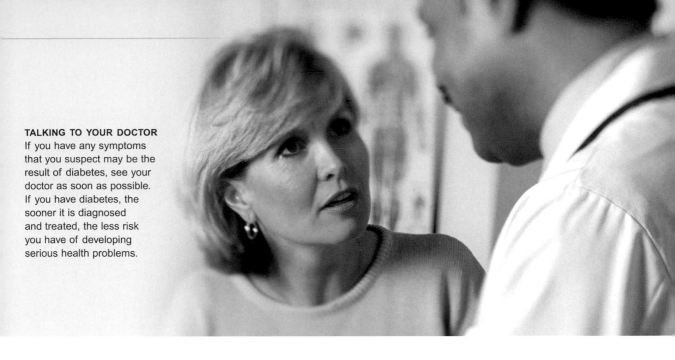

TALKING TO YOUR DOCTOR
If you have any symptoms
that you suspect may be the
result of diabetes, see your
doctor as soon as possible.
If you have diabetes, the
sooner it is diagnosed
and treated, the less risk
you have of developing
serious health problems.

day-to-day activities, and still feel
tired even if you rest or sleep more
than usual. This is because some or
all of the glucose in your blood
cannot enter your body cells to give
you energy.

■ **WEIGHT LOSS** When your body
cannot use glucose, it starts to break
down its fat and muscle stores for
energy instead, so you may lose
weight. Weight loss is more common
and rapid in Type 1 than Type 2
diabetes. In Type 2, weight loss may
happen very slowly or not at all.

If you are overweight, you may be
pleased to lose weight in such an
effortless way. This isn't healthy,
however, and, as soon as your diabetes
is under control, you should expect to
regain the weight that you have lost.

■ **BLURRED VISION** When your blood
glucose level is high, the lenses of
your eyes absorb glucose and water.
This makes them swell, which
causes blurred vision.

■ **FRUITY-SMELLING BREATH** This is a
late symptom of Type 1 diabetes and
indicates a dangerously high blood
glucose level. When your body
breaks down fat for energy it
produces toxic by-products called
ketones. If your breath smells
fruity (the smell is often said to
be similar to that of pear drops or
nail varnish remover), this is a sign
that your body is trying to expel
ketones via your lungs. If you also
develop any of the following
symptoms: nausea, vomiting,
and/or abdominal pain, you may
need urgent hospital treatment for
ketoacidosis (diabetic coma), which
although rare, can be extremely
dangerous (see p.113).

■ **THRUSH AND CYSTITIS** The presence
of glucose in your urine provides
a good environment for bacteria
and germs to grow in large
amounts, making infections such
as cystitis and thrush more likely.

Fruity-smelling
breath is a late
symptom of
Type 1 diabetes
and indicates a
dangerously
high blood
glucose level.

MEDICAL TESTS USED IN THE DIAGNOSIS OF DIABETES

Although urine and fingerprick tests can reveal a higher than normal blood glucose level, you need one or more of three laboratory blood tests to diagnose diabetes: the random or fasting blood glucose test and, if necessary, the oral glucose tolerance test. Your results are assessed with your symptoms. If you don't have symptoms but diabetes is suspected, you need a repeat blood test carried out on a different day.

HOW THE TEST IS CARRIED OUT	WHAT THE RESULTS MEAN
Urine test 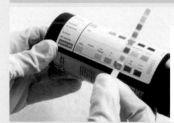 A health professional tests a sample of your urine using a dipstick that changes colour according to the amount of glucose present. The dipstick is then compared to a colour chart. A result is obtained within 1 minute.	The presence or absence of glucose in urine does not necessarily indicate or discount diabetes. If your urine contains glucose, or you have symptoms but no glucose, you will be referred for further blood tests.
Fingerprick test 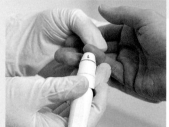 A health professional uses a device to prick the side of your fingertip and puts a drop of blood from your finger onto a testing strip. This strip is then inserted in a blood glucose meter in the surgery to be analysed. A result is obtained within 1 minute.	A healthy blood glucose level is in the range of 4–6 millimoles per litre. If your test result is above 6 millimoles per litre, your health professional will ask you to have further blood tests. A fingerprick test by itself is not enough to diagnose diabetes.
Random blood glucose test 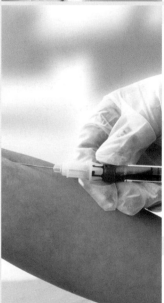 Your health professional takes a blood sample from your arm to send to a laboratory for analysis. This sample can be taken regardless of whether you have eaten. Your health professional receives the results within a week.	If you have symptoms and a test result above 11.1 millimoles per litre, you are diagnosed with diabetes. If you have no symptoms, or the result is less than this, you may repeat the test while fasting or take an oral glucose tolerance test.
Fasting blood glucose test You do not eat or drink overnight and in the morning your health professional takes a blood sample from your arm. The sample is sent to a laboratory for analysis. Your health professional receives the results within a week.	If you have symptoms and a test result above 7 millimoles per litre, you have diabetes. If you have no symptoms, or the result is less than this and you have symptoms, you may repeat the test or take an oral glucose tolerance test.
Oral glucose tolerance test You do not eat or drink overnight and in the morning your health professional takes a blood sample from your arm before and 2 hours after drinking some glucose. The samples are sent for analysis. Your health professional usually receives the results in a week.	If your fasting level is above 7 millimoles per litre and/or your 2 hour test result is above 11.1 millimoles per litre, you are diagnosed with diabetes, whether or not you have symptoms. This test is used when other tests have been inconclusive or to diagnose gestational diabetes.

Diagnosing diabetes

Diabetes must be diagnosed by a blood test in which a blood sample is analysed in a laboratory (see opposite). Type 1 diabetes is likely to be diagnosed more quickly than Type 2, because the symptoms usually develop rapidly and are more severe. Type 2 diabetes is sometimes suspected when you are showing early signs of complications. For example, abnormal changes at the back of your eye may be noticed at a routine eye examination.

Your diabetes will be diagnosed by one or more of three blood tests: a random blood glucose test, a fasting blood glucose test, and an oral glucose tolerance test. Tests such as fingerprick and urine tests are not sufficient to confirm or discount the presence of diabetes (see opposite). If your fasting blood glucose level is 6–7 millimoles per litre, your blood glucose is not normal, but not high enough for diabetes to be diagnosed. Your health professional will explain what your test results mean and the implications they have for you.

Medical tests after diagnosis

One of the main aims of diabetes care is to prevent long-term complications, so within about three months of diagnosis, you will be offered the following routine tests to check your general health and for signs that any complications may be developing. Your test results form the starting point for your yearly check-up, known as your annual review

---

My experience

> *"I remember being told I had diabetes but I had no idea of what that actually meant."* SOPHIE

COMMENT Anxiety, fear, disbelief, and denial are common reactions at diagnosis. If it helps, talk to your health professional about these feelings. After the shock it's common to want to learn as much as you can about diabetes management so you can incorporate diabetes care into your life.

(see p.26). If any problems are discovered, you will be referred for the appropriate treatment.

■ **HEIGHT, WEIGHT AND BODY MASS INDEX** Your body mass index (BMI) is calculated (see p.46). Your BMI shows whether or not you are overweight for your height.

■ **BLOOD PRESSURE** High blood pressure is particularly common in people with Type 2 diabetes. If your blood pressure is high over a period of time, you will be prescribed medication to lower it.

■ **FOOT EXAMINATION** A health professional checks your foot circulation and nerve supply and teaches you how to look after your own feet (see pp.128–130).

■ **EYE EXAMINATION** The retina at the back of your eye is checked for damaged blood vessels either by using an instrument known as an ophthalmoscope or an eye camera.

■ **OTHER TESTS** Blood tests are performed to check kidney, liver, and thyroid function, and blood fat levels. An HbA1c test measures your glucose level over the previous six to eight weeks (see p.23). Your urine is tested for protein (a possible sign of early kidney damage; see pp.196–199).

Type 1 diabetes is likely to be diagnosed more quickly than Type 2 because the symptoms usually develop rapidly and are more severe.

Looking after your diabetes

If you look after yourself and your diabetes, you can continue to live life to the full. Regularly testing your blood glucose level, eating and drinking healthily, doing plenty of physical activity, and taking your tablets and/or insulin injections all help you to control your blood glucose level effectively. Good blood glucose control is vital to reduce your risk of developing long-term complications, and your health professional works with you to achieve this.

Monitoring blood glucose

When you have diabetes, your body cannot control your blood glucose level in the usual way. The key to caring for your diabetes is to keep your blood glucose level within the recommended range of 4–7 millimoles per litre. Monitoring your blood glucose level regularly and adjusting your treatment accordingly will help you to achieve this. This is critical in the prevention of long-term complications (see pp.26–27).

My experience

"The more you know about diabetes, the better you can control it and the more flexible you can be. That message has informed my life." JOE

COMMENT Learning as much as you can about diabetes can help you to fit it into your life. Also, blood glucose monitoring helps you learn about how different situations affect your blood glucose level. Your test results enable you to make informed decisions about how to control your diabetes.

Home testing

Measuring your own blood glucose is easier and more accurate than ever before. There is a huge range of testing equipment available, from basic blood testing strips to sophisticated electronic meters with computer download facilities that allow you to analyse the results (see pp.67–70).

When and how often you test your blood glucose largely depends on your treatment, the food you eat, and your physical activity. The aim is to find a time and frequency to suit you and to give you the information you need to control your diabetes effectively. For a step-by-step guide to blood glucose testing see pp.62–75.

Whatever type of diabetes you have, the recommended blood glucose level to aim for is 4–7 millimoles per litre. This is close enough to the normal range of people who don't have diabetes, to reduce the risk of possible long-term complications.

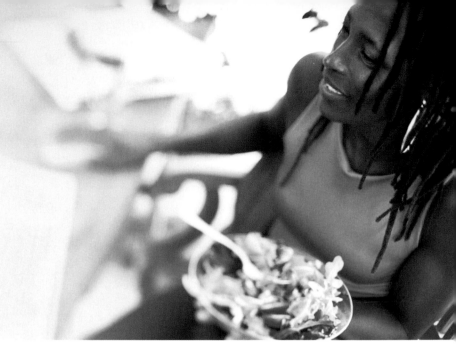

The HbA1c test

Although testing your blood glucose level at home is a key part of diabetes care there is another type of blood glucose test called the HbA1c test, which is carried out by a health professional at least once or twice a year. The difference between this and your home tests is that the latter give day-to-day readings of your blood glucose level and the HbA1c test gives an overall measure of your blood glucose level for the previous six to eight weeks. HbA1c results are given as a percentage – the closer they are to 7 per cent (or below) the better.

Controlling blood glucose

Keeping your blood glucose level well controlled is one of the most effective actions you can take to prevent long-term complications and keep you feeling well. Good control means that

Q What does it mean if my HbA1c result is above 7 per cent?

A It means that you should discuss your diabetes management with your health professional. Even a result of 7.5 per cent is considered to be unsatisfactory control of diabetes. For every 1 per cent rise in your HbA1c result, there is a 30 per cent increase in the likelihood of you developing complications affecting your blood vessels and nerves, so being strict about a 7 per cent result is important.

the majority of your home blood glucose test results fall within the range of 4–7 millimoles per litre. This means that your HbA1c result will be close to 7 per cent. The four main factors that affect your blood glucose control are food and drink, physical activity, tablets, and insulin injections. When your blood glucose level is poorly controlled you will experience hypoglycaemia (low blood glucose) or hyperglycaemia (high blood glucose).

Good control means that the majority of your home blood test results fall within the range of 4–7 millimoles per litre.

Practical tips

KEEPING YOUR BLOOD GLUCOSE CONTROLLED

• Eat regular, healthy meals to avoid major fluctuations in your blood glucose level.

• Stay physically active to help your insulin work more efficiently.

• Maintain your weight in the recommended range, both to avoid needing large amounts of insulin and to reduce your risk of heart disease.

• Take any diabetes tablets or insulin you have been prescribed every day.

• Monitor your blood glucose level closely and learn to adjust your treatment to the results.

If your blood glucose level gets very low, less glucose reaches your brain, making concentration difficult.

■ **FOOD AND DRINK** Eating regular meals based on carbohydrates throughout the day helps you to avoid major fluctuations in your blood glucose level. If you have Type 2 diabetes, attention to what you eat combined with physical activity may be enough to keep your blood glucose well controlled for several years. If you take tablets and/or inject insulin, you may sometimes need to alter your eating pattern to suit the timing or dose of your treatment. (For more information on healthy eating and drinking, see pp.30–43.)

■ **PHYSICAL ACTIVITY** Keeping physically active helps you to control your blood glucose level by improving your body's sensitivity to insulin. Regular activity helps to lower your blood glucose level and keep it better controlled in the long term. If you take tablets or inject insulin, you need to be aware that physical activity can reduce your blood glucose level in a short time. You may need to alter your treatment accordingly. (For more information on this and physical activity, see pp.52–59.)

■ **TABLETS** You may need to take tablets to control your blood glucose level if you have Type 2 diabetes. Tablets work by increasing the amount of insulin you produce, by helping body cells to use insulin more effectively, or by slowing down carbohydrate digestion. You and your health professional can discuss which tablets are likely to best control your diabetes. (For more information on tablets, see pp.76–81.)

■ **INSULIN INJECTIONS** If you have Type 1 diabetes, you need insulin injections to control your blood glucose level. If you have Type 2 diabetes you may also need insulin injections. There are various types of insulin, all of which are active for different lengths of time: some act within 5 minutes and wear off within 4 hours; others keep working for 24 hours or longer. Your health professional works with you to decide which type of insulin is best for you (see pp.82–101).

Hypoglycaemia

If you take insulin or insulin-stimulating tablets, your blood glucose level may sometimes fall below 4 millimoles per litre, This is referred to as hypoglycaemia, or a "hypo". Reasons for hypoglycaemia include:

• Taking too high a dose of diabetes medication, or the wrong sort of medication for you.

• Being more active than usual.

• Missing or delaying meals.

• Drinking too much alcohol without compensating with food.

• Taking insulin-stimulating tablets together with other drugs, such as co-trimoxazole, trimethoprim (antibacterials), monoamineoxidase inhibitors (a type of antidepressant), and ranitidine (an anti-ulcer drug).

• Other conditions, such as underactive thyroid or reduced kidney function, which mean that insulin or tablets are not excreted efficiently.

The main symptoms of a hypo are feeling shaky, sweaty, hungry, and getting pins and needles in your lips, but the symptoms vary from person to person. If your blood glucose level gets very low (below 2.5 millimoles per litre), less glucose reaches your brain, making concentration difficult. People may notice that you are acting strangely. For example, you might struggle to carry out a simple task or your speech might be slurred.

If you feel a hypo coming on, you need to eat or drink something that quickly raises your blood glucose level, such as glucose tablets, a glucose drink, or sugar lumps. If you are confused because your blood glucose is very low, you may need other people's help to take something. This is why it can be useful to tell friends and colleagues that you have diabetes. If your hypo is not treated, you may lose consciousness. (For more about hypos, see pp.102–109).

Hyperglycaemia

A high level of glucose in your blood is referred to as hyperglycaemia. If your blood glucose level rises above the recommended 7 millimoles per litre but is below 10 millimoles per litre, you are likely to still feel well. Above this level, however, the symptoms of hyperglycaemia start to appear. Although mild and temporary hyperglycaemia won't damage your body, a high blood glucose level over months or years can lead to long-term complications of diabetes. Reasons for hyperglycaemia include:
● Not taking enough medication to lower your blood glucose level, either because you are on too low a dose

My experience

"There's a tension between knowing I must look after my diabetes and feeling determined not to let it stop me from doing anything I want." JOE

COMMENT If you feel that diabetes dominates your life and prevents you from doing things, you might be less motivated to manage your condition effectively. Talk to your health professional about ways of integrating your treatment into your daily routine.

or because you haven't been able to take it regularly.
● Being less active than usual.
● Eating very large meals or lots of high-sugar foods.
● Being ill.

The symptoms of hyperglycaemia include passing large amounts of urine, intense thirst, fatigue, and infections, such as thrush and cystitis – the same symptoms that may have prompted you to seek treatment before you were diagnosed with diabetes. If your blood glucose level continues to rise and you have Type 1 diabetes, you may develop diabetic ketoacidosis (see p.113); if you have Type 2 diabetes, you may develop excessive dehydration, which may lead to coma, known as non-ketotic hyperosmolar state (see p.113). Both need hospital treatment. For more about hyperglycaemia, see pp.110–13.

If you frequently have a low or high blood glucose level or swing between the two, the type, quantity, or timing of your medication, physical activity, or eating may need to change. Your health professional can discuss causes of hypoglycaemia and hyperglycaemia and suggest appropriate action.

Myth OR
TRUTH?

MYTH
If I feel well, my blood glucose level must be well controlled.

TRUTH
You can feel well and still have a high blood glucose level, particularly if your body has become used to it being high – not everyone has symptoms. The best way to know your blood glucose level is to test regularly.

Working with your health professional

Treatment and care for your diabetes is individually tailored to you, based on the type of diabetes you have and how well controlled your blood glucose level and other aspects of your health are. One of the most important aspects of your medical care is your annual diabetes review.

The annual review

At your annual review, your health professional assesses how well your blood glucose level is controlled and checks for any signs of the long-term complications of diabetes. You have the same routine tests that were carried out shortly after your diagnosis (see p.21). Tests for long-term complications are described in detail on pp.186–215.

It is important to recognize that your annual review should be an exchange of information and it's fine to offer your own ideas about diabetes

management (see pp.148–151). Your health professional can offer both medical and psychological help and can:

- Give you information about your type of diabetes.
- Explain how your treatment works and whether you need any changes to your treatment.
- Listen and support you if you are finding it difficult to stay motivated about managing your diabetes.
- Discuss the implications of your diabetes on your work, family, and social life, and help you to work out how to overcome potential problems.
- Provide information about how often you need appointments with a health professional and how you can get in touch between visits.
- Explain which other health professionals you might need to see and why.
- Ensure you have a written record of plans made during your visit.

It's often necessary to see your diabetes health professional more than once a year. This may be related to changes in your treatment, problems with a high or low blood glucose level, or because you need to review other aspects of your care.

Long-term complications

The complications of diabetes can cause damage slowly over a period of years without any sign that they are doing so. Complications are largely caused by a consistently high

ANNUAL REVIEW
As well as assessing your blood glucose level and general health, your annual review gives you the opportunity to discuss any day-to-day problems you might have with managing your diabetes.

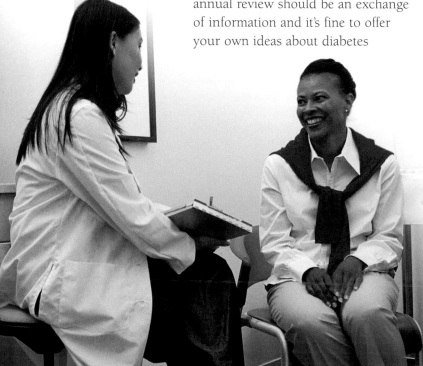

blood glucose level, which slowly damages your blood circulation and nerves over years. If you have Type 1 diabetes, you are unlikely to develop any complications within the first 10 years of diagnosis. The length of time before complications develop in Type 2 varies. Because Type 2 diabetes can go unnoticed for many years, you may have complications at the time you are diagnosed. (For more information on long-term complications, see pp.148–151.)

Types of long-term complication

Having diabetes makes you more susceptible to a number of health conditions such as:

■ **DEPRESSION** Day-to-day pressures of living with diabetes (and anticipating possible long-term complications) may have psychological effects (see pp.186–189).

■ **EYE CONDITIONS** Damage can occur to the blood vessels that supply blood to the retina at the back of your eye, leading to impaired vision. Cataracts are also more common when you have diabetes (see pp.190–195).

■ **KIDNEY CONDITIONS** Gradual damage to the kidneys' filtering system may eventually lead to kidney failure (see pp.196–199).

■ **FOOT CONDITIONS** Poor circulation and damage to nerves can lead to a loss of sensation in your feet and problems such as ulcers, damage to the bones of the foot, and even gangrene (see pp.200–205).

My experience

"I am frightened about long-term complications – it's the unknown – but my annual checks give me an objective view of my diabetes." STUART

COMMENT The key to preventing long-term complications is to ensure that your blood glucose level is well controlled as much of the time as possible. At your annual review you are checked for signs of long-term complications and referred for treatment if necessary.

■ **CARDIOVASCULAR CONDITIONS** Conditions include high blood pressure, hyperlipidaemia, coronary heart disease, stroke, and peripheral vascular disease (see pp.206–211).

■ **OTHER CONDITIONS** Injecting can cause skin conditions, and damage to the nervous and circulatory systems can cause erectile dysfunction and autonomic neuropathy (see pp.212–215).

Preventing complications

Because the long-term complications of diabetes are largely caused by too much glucose in your blood over a long period of time, any improvement you make in controlling blood glucose is beneficial. Eating healthily, being physically active, losing weight if you need to, and stopping smoking, also greatly reduce your risk of developing complications. It is also important to check your feet daily (see pp.128–130) and seek help if you notice any injuries or abnormalities. Other actions that improve your control are taking your daily tablets and/or insulin correctly, attending your annual review and keeping your knowledge of diabetes up-to-date.

Complications of diabetes can cause damage slowly over a period of years without any sign that they are doing so.

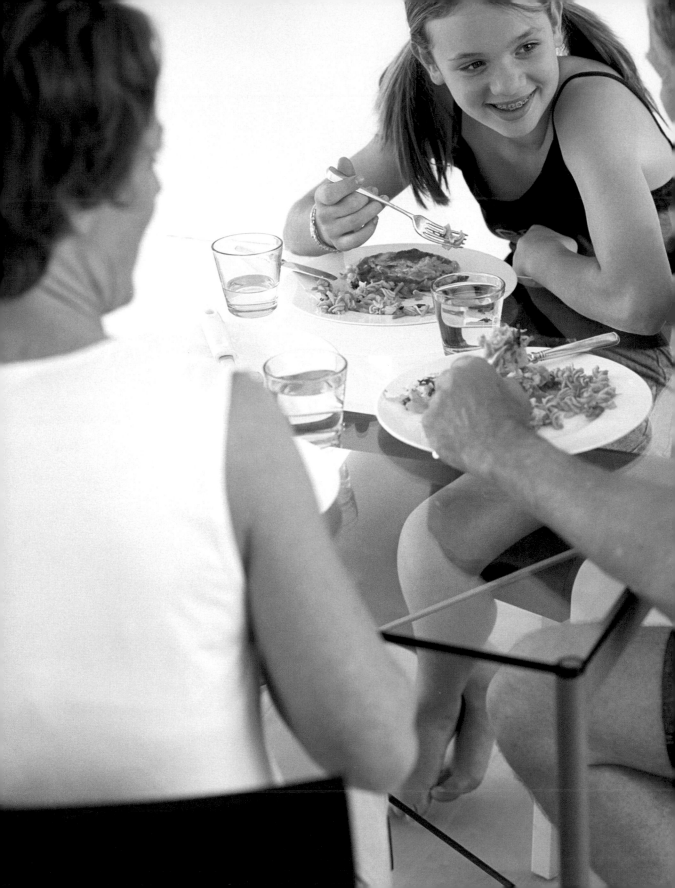

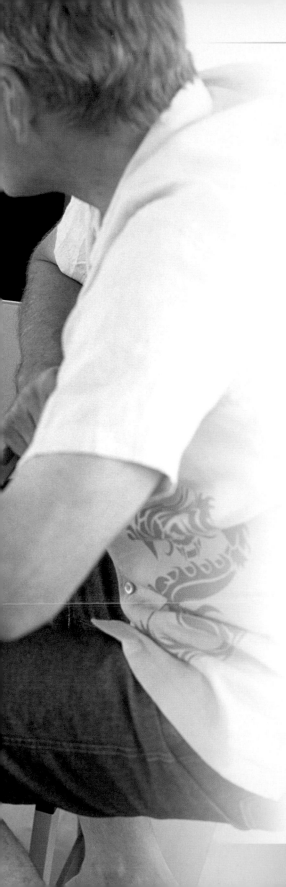

Food, drink, and physical activity

The guidelines for healthy eating and drinking and being active apply to everyone, but are especially important if you have diabetes. If you have Type 2 diabetes, you may be able to manage your condition effectively with food, drink, and physical activity. If you take insulin or tablets for your diabetes, you can also influence your blood glucose level by using the information in this chapter.

There are compelling health reasons for taking steps to prevent weight gain and obesity when you have diabetes. If you are overweight, losing weight can make a big difference to how well your blood glucose level is controlled.

Becoming more active can also help you to lose weight. In addition, regular physical activity has benefits for your overall health and wellbeing, as well as your diabetes. And by being aware of the impact that physical activity has on your blood glucose level, you will be able to adjust your diabetes treatment if necessary.

Healthy eating and drinking

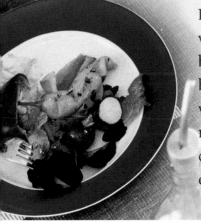

Having diabetes is about making healthy eating choices whenever you can, eating regularly – or at the right times to balance the effects of any tablets and/or insulin you take – and being aware of the effects of alcohol on your diabetes. Knowing what's in your food – carbohydrates, protein, fat, vitamins, minerals, and fibre – enables you to make choices that help to control your blood glucose level. Whether you cook at home or eat out, there are ways to enjoy food and care for your diabetes.

You need to eat carbohydrate-containing foods because they are your body's main source of energy, but choosing those that have less immediate effect on blood glucose helps your body deal with them.

Healthy eating principles

The principles of healthy eating for people with diabetes are the same as those for everyone else. No foods are banned – but some should be eaten less often. Sometimes you don't have a choice about what food is available, but generally you can adapt recipes and meals so that you can enjoy food while eating healthily. The principles of healthy eating are as follows:

- Eat regular meals that contain carbohydrate.
- Eat more high-fibre foods, including fruit and vegetables (at least 5 portions per day).
- Choose wholegrain foods if possible.
- Cut down on fat.
- Eat red meat in moderation.
- Limit added sugar/sugary foods.
- Reduce your salt intake.
- Keep your alcohol consumption to the recommended limits.

Food and diabetes

When you have diabetes, your body is unable to use foods that contain carbohydrate in the usual way. All foods containing carbohydrate are broken down into glucose. You need insulin to let glucose into your cells for energy now, as well as to store some glucose in your liver for energy later. Because you have less insulin available or your insulin is not working effectively, your blood glucose level will rise when you eat carbohydrates and remain high. You still need to eat

Q Will I need to follow a "diabetic diet"?

A No – there is no such thing as a diabetic diet. In fact, the basic principles of healthy eating for people with diabetes are the same as the recommendations for everyone else. You certainly don't need to follow any restrictive meal plans or eat products labelled as "diabetic".

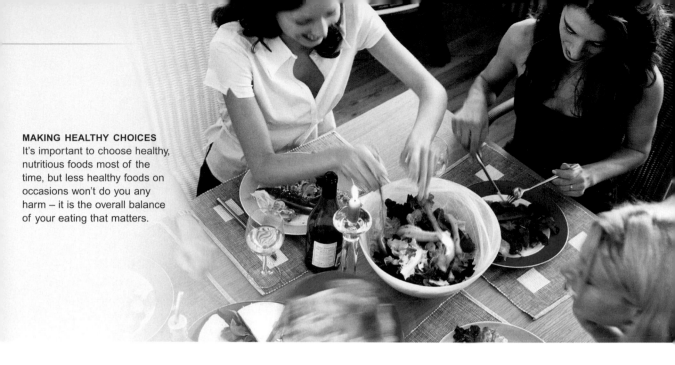

MAKING HEALTHY CHOICES
It's important to choose healthy, nutritious foods most of the time, but less healthy foods on occasions won't do you any harm – it is the overall balance of your eating that matters.

carbohydrate-containing foods because they are your body's main source of energy, but choosing those that have less immediate effect on your blood glucose level, and eating them in amounts that will balance with any tablets and/or insulin you take, will help your body to deal with them.

■ **TYPE 1 DIABETES** If you have Type 1 diabetes, matching your food intake to the action of your insulin is the way to maintain a healthy blood glucose level. For example, if you take a shorter-acting insulin, you will need to take it around the time that you are having your meals. You will also be taking a longer-acting insulin, and you may need to eat extra snacks to make sure that there is food available in your body when your insulin is working at its peak. The exact timing of your food and insulin together will depend on the type of insulin you take (see pp.82–101).

■ **TYPE 2 DIABETES** If you have Type 2 diabetes, your body's ability to produce insulin effectively when you eat is impaired, so eating foods that take longer to be broken down into glucose can help your pancreas to cope. Sugary foods are converted into glucose fastest so eating them after a meal, when your body is already slowly digesting other food, can help to reduce their impact on your blood glucose. Also, avoiding eating a lot of carbohydrate-containing food at once helps to reduce the pressure on your pancreas to produce large amounts of insulin.

If you are taking tablets for your diabetes, you will need to take them in relation to your meals. This is because some work by helping your body to break down food more slowly, and others make your pancreas produce more insulin, so if they are not timed correctly with

My experience

"For years, the type of insulin I took dictated when I had to eat because if I didn't eat, I would go hypo. Now, with newer insulins and delivery mechanisms, I can match my insulin to when I want to eat." STUART

COMMENT If you are finding it difficult to eat at the right times to match your insulin, you may be able to try one of the many new insulins available. The latest insulins cause fewer hypos and enable you to eat what, when, and how much you want. Ask your health professional for advice.

If your routine is unpredictable or your usual eating pattern is disrupted, you may find that your blood glucose level is less well controlled.

meals they will not be effective and may cause hypoglycaemia (see pp.102–109).

It is common to be overweight if you have Type 2 diabetes, so you may also need to look at eating with a view to losing weight (see pp.44–51 for more information). Having Type 2 diabetes in particular is linked with an increased risk of developing high blood pressure, high cholesterol, and circulatory disease, and eating healthily can help to reduce this risk.

Food, drink, and your day

An important part of your diabetes control is recognizing when you need to eat or drink in order to balance the effects of tablets or insulin on your blood glucose level. If your routine is unpredictable, or your usual eating pattern is disrupted, you may find that your blood glucose level is less well controlled.

If you take insulin or tablets to stimulate your insulin production (see pp.76–101), eating at regular intervals throughout the day is essential to avoid hypos. If you inject insulin or take tablets to increase the insulin in your bloodstream and you don't eat, your blood glucose level will fall. There are some tablets (see pp.76–81) and insulins (see pp.82–101) now available that enable you to closely match your insulin to your food, making it less likely that you will have too much insulin in your bloodstream.

Regularly eating meals containing carbohydrate throughout the day will "fuel" your body, help your digestive system to function properly, and avoid sharp rises and falls in your blood glucose level. If you have only one large meal a day, your body will struggle to turn this into energy quickly enough to keep your blood glucose level balanced. A regular eating

Q I am vegetarian and I'm also Muslim, so I sometimes fast for religious reasons. How do I cope with this and with my diabetes?

A The healthy eating principles remain the same whether you are vegetarian or are following any other special diet – for example if you eat kosher food, or if you have coeliac disease or allergies to certain foods. If you find it difficult to find enough variety of foods to eat, you can seek professional dietary advice. When you fast, you may need to adjust the dosage of your tablets or insulin for the period that you are fasting and the times that you eat. Ask your health professional for guidance. In general, fasting during pregnancy when you have diabetes is not recommended as it can be harmful to you and your unborn child.

pattern is also more likely to fit in with any tablets or insulin you take for your diabetes.

■ **TIMING YOUR FOOD WITH MEDICATION**
Knowing when your tablets or insulin will work and when your blood glucose level is likely to start falling is useful. For example, some tablets may make your blood glucose level fall mid-morning or mid-afternoon, in which case you might need to eat a snack at these times. If you can't eat when you need to, perhaps because of long shifts or meetings at work, for example, you may need a different medication that will suit your routine better. Discuss this with your health professional.

■ **SNACKING** Having diabetes does not automatically mean having to add snacks to your day – it may be that eating regular meals at certain times controls your blood glucose level well enough. Also, if you are trying to lose weight, you may not want to increase your calorie intake. However, if you are taking certain types of insulin or tablets, you may need snacks between meals and before bed to keep your blood glucose level steady. Or you may simply want a snack because you are hungry. If this is the case, try to make sure snacks are not all high in fat or sugar – a piece of fruit instead of a biscuit is much healthier. Also, snacking should not mean you eat more food overall – by reducing what you eat at other times, such as by having smaller meals, snacks will not be extras but part of your normal daily food intake.

Food groups

Foods fall into three main groups: carbohydrates, proteins, and fats. Eating the right balance of foods from each of these groups on a daily basis will help keep you healthy. You also need to be aware of the fruit and vegetables, vitamins and minerals, fibre, and salt that you are eating. Finally, you need to know the sugar content of different drinks. Once you have a clear idea of which types of food are better for you and in what quantities, shopping, cooking, and choosing meals when you are out will be far easier.

Carbohydrates

Carbohydrates fall into two categories: "simple carbohydrates", which are also known as sugars, and "complex carbohydrates", known as starches.

■ **SIMPLE CARBOHYDRATES** These are sugars in their simplest form (also known as sucrose or glucose). Foods that are high in sugar include sweets, chocolate, sugary drinks, and some cakes. Because sugars are made up of only a few molecules, they are digested easily and rapidly, causing your blood glucose level to rise sharply – creating an immediate demand for more insulin. For this reason, you should eat these foods in small quantities, and preferably with or after other food, to slow down their absorption. However, you don't need to avoid sugar completely. This would be very difficult, because it is a hidden ingredient in many foods. Checking food labels and choosing

SIMPLE CARBOHYDRATES
Some cakes and pastries contain simple carbohydrates, and when you eat these foods your blood glucose will rise sharply.

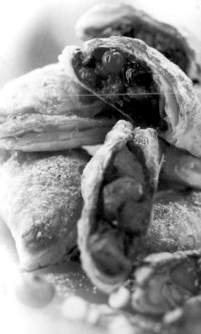

foods with a lower sugar content will help to keep your blood glucose level better controlled.

■ **COMPLEX CARBOHYDRATES** These include bread, potatoes, rice, pasta, cereals, and beans and pulses. They are broken down into glucose, but are digested relatively slowly so, unlike simple carbohydrates, they do not raise blood glucose dramatically.

GLYCAEMIC INDEX OF COMMON FOODS

Foods are given a GI number between 1 and 100, with glucose (sugar) scoring 100 because it causes blood glucose to rise very quickly – within 30 minutes of being eaten. Different foods need to be specifically measured for their GI rating, and individual brands of the same food can vary. The following are guidelines.

LOW (below 55)	MEDIUM (55–70)	HIGH (over 70)
Apples	Melons	Dates
Bananas	Pineapples	Watermelons
Carrots	Beetroot	Swede
Tomatoes	Sweetcorn	Parsnips
Porridge with milk	Muesli	Cornflakes
Rolled oats	Instant porridge	Puffed rice cereal
Oat bran	Grape nuts	Wheat biscuit cereal
Granary bread	Wholemeal bread	Brown bread
Mixed grain bread	Rye bread	White bread
Pitta bread	Croissants	Bagels
Pasta	Brown rice	Instant rice
Instant noodles	Couscous	Mashed potatoes
Sweet potatoes	New potatoes	Baked potatoes
Crisps	Muffins	Rice cakes
Peanuts	Digestive biscuits	Wafer biscuits
Popcorn	Muesli bars	Doughnuts
Orange juice	Cranberry juice	Glucose drink
Yoghurt	Full-fat ice-cream	Tapioca

Managing your carbohydrate intake

Knowing how much carbohydrate is contained in what you eat and how quickly particular foods will cause your blood glucose level to rise helps you to manage the amount and types of food you eat. There are two common ways of managing your carbohydrate intake: the glycaemic index and carbohydrate counting.

The glycaemic index

The glycaemic index (GI) is a ranking of carbohydrate-containing foods based on their effect on your blood glucose level. Foods that are digested slowly have a low GI rating and foods that are quickly absorbed have a high rating. The index is useful because you can help to keep your blood glucose level in the recommended range by monitoring the GI rating of your food. If you eat too many high GI foods, your blood glucose level rises sharply and falls quickly. For this reason, eating more low and medium GI foods than high ones balances your blood glucose level.

However, the GI of a particular food only tells you how quickly or slowly it raises blood glucose when eaten on its own. You usually eat a mixture of foods at any one meal – bread is often eaten with butter or margarine, and potatoes with meat and vegetables, for example. Combining foods with different GI ratings changes the overall GI of meal. Therefore, the way to use the GI is as a guide to what low GI foods to include in a meal or snack to lower the overall effect on your blood glucose level. If you eat a baked potato (high GI), for example, adding baked beans (low GI) reduces the overall GI of the meal, as well as helping to balance your meal.

It's also important not to confine yourself solely to low GI foods: this could lead to more hypos, especially if you are taking tablets or insulin, because this might result in you having more insulin in your system than you need. Some low GI foods are also higher in fat – peanuts, for example – so they are not the best choice if you want to eat healthily.

Carbohydrate counting

Carbohydrate (CHO) counting is a way of assessing how much carbohydrate you are eating so that you can calculate how much insulin you need. If you were diagnosed with diabetes in the 1980s, you may have been taught CHO counting as a method of blood glucose control. At that time, it was thought that if you ate similar amounts of carbohydrate at set times each day, your blood glucose level would be the same every day. But CHO counting in this way wasn't very effective and meant restricting your food intake to match your insulin, so it is no longer popular.

Today, CHO counting is being used in conjunction with newer rapid-acting insulins to give people more freedom about what they eat. It is most valuable if you have Type 1 diabetes because you choose what to

UNDERSTANDING CARBOHYDRATE CONTENT

The more carbohydrate your food contains, the more insulin you need to convert it into energy. Knowing how much carbohydrate is in different foods can help you adjust your medication to deal with it.

AMOUNT	TYPE OF CARBOHYDRATE
10g CHO	1 thin slice bread, 1 tablespoon uncooked rice, 1 digestive biscuit, 2 tablespoons baked beans, 1 small apple
15g CHO	1 medium slice bread, 1 90g boiled potato, 7–10 medium chips, 1 crumpet, 1 medium sausage roll, 1 medium grapefruit
20g CHO	1 thick slice bread, 1 large croissant, 1 cup custard, 1 mango, 2 tablespoons raisins
30g CHO	1 bagel, 1 large scone, 1 cup bran cereal, 1 jam tart, 4 slices pineapple, 8–10 dried apricots

eat and then match your quick- or rapid-acting insulin doses, via injection or insulin pump, to the amount of CHO the food contains.

To establish your personal quick- or rapid-acting insulin to carbohydrate ratio, you need to find out how much insulin you need for every 10g of CHO (for example) you eat. If, for example, you need 1 unit of insulin for every 10g of carbohydrate, your

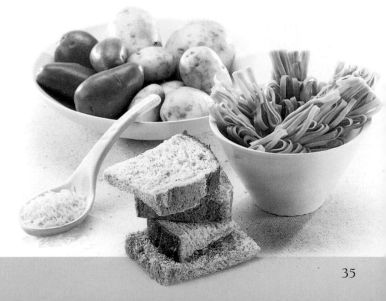

COMPLEX CARBOHYDRATES
You should aim to include complex carbohydrates in every meal to give you a sustained supply of energy without overloading your system at any one time.

ratio will be 1 unit to 10g CHO. You can then use this to calculate how much insulin you need whenever you eat any carbohydrate-containing food.

If you are finding it difficult to control your blood glucose and you are prepared to carry out more frequent blood glucose testing and assess your food and insulin doses throughout each day, your health professional can help you to find out more about using this method.

Proteins

Protein-rich foods include meat, fish, eggs, cheese, beans, and pulses. Your body needs protein to create, maintain and repair its cells but to eat healthily, protein should make up only about a fifth of any meal. Protein has little effect on your blood glucose level but when you are choosing which type of protein to eat, you can make healthier choices – for example by ensuring that you do not eat red meat every day, or that you eat reduced-fat cheese, and include fish in your meal 2–3 times a week.

Fats

Fats are found in dairy products, such as milk, butter, and cheese, cooking oils, meats, and nuts, as well as in processed foods. Everyone needs to eat a small amount of fat – it is an important component of many body cells and plays a key role in growth and development. However, it is recommended that women should eat no more than 70g of fat per day, and men no more than 95g per day. The type of fat you eat is also important.

Fats have little effect on blood glucose but there are good reasons to limit your fat intake when you have diabetes. Eating too much fat is linked to high levels of fat in the blood (hyperlipidaemia), heart and

---

DIFFERENT TYPES OF FAT

Some types of fats are better for you than others, so it's useful to know which increase your chances of developing heart and circulatory problems and which (in small quantities) are beneficial to your health.

HEALTHIER FATS

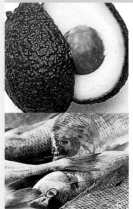

MONOUNSATURATED FATS Found in some margarines and cooking oils, including olive oil and canola or rapeseed oil, and also in avocados, nuts, and seeds, these fats do not raise cholesterol levels (and are even thought to lower them). They are a healthier alternative to saturated fats (see below).

POLYUNSATURATED FATS There are two groups of polyunsaturated fatty acids, omega-3 and omega-6. Omega-3 is found in oily fish, rapeseed oil, and walnuts. Omega-6 is found in sunflower, safflower, and corn oils. Like monounsaturated fats, they are healthier than saturated fats.

LESS HEALTHY FATS

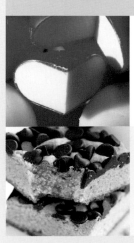

SATURATED FATS These are mainly found in animal products – butter, cheese, and the fat around a piece of steak are examples – but they are also found in coconut and palm oils. These fats raise blood cholesterol, which can lead to health problems including high blood pressure and heart disease.

TRANS FATTY ACIDS Often listed on food labels as "hydrogenated" or "partially hydrogenated" these synthetic saturated fatty acids are in many processed foods, such as biscuits and cakes. They raise cholesterol levels, and eating foods that are high in trans fatty acids is linked to an increased risk of a heart attack.

circulatory disease, and stroke (see pp.206–211) – all complications of diabetes. Being overweight can also contribute to the risk of developing these complications, and fats are very high in calories. While dairy products are high in fat, they also contain protein and carbohydrate and are a source of calcium and vitamins. To protect against heart and circulatory conditions, and also to help if you are trying to lose weight, choose lower-fat versions of fatty foods, such as skimmed or semi-skimmed instead of full-fat milk.

Vitamins and minerals

A healthy, balanced food intake provides all the vitamins and minerals you need. Whether you have diabetes or not, you do not need to take vitamin or mineral supplements unless your doctor or health professional advises it. Research suggests that anti-oxidants, including beta-carotene, vitamin E, and lipoic acid may help to counteract insulin resistance and protect against heart and circulatory conditions.

Fruit and vegetables

As well as being low in calories and rich in fibre, fruit and vegetables are excellent sources of vitamins and minerals. To eat healthily, your daily food intake should include at least five portions of fruit and vegetables – fresh, tinned (in natural juice or water rather than syrup), frozen, or dried. A portion is one piece of fruit such as an apple or pear, a 150ml glass of fruit juice, 3 tablespoons of vegetables, or a small salad. However, fruit and natural fruit juices also contain sugar (fructose), so more than one piece of fruit at a time, or more than a small glass of fruit juice a day will raise your blood glucose level. Space out your fruit consumption throughout the day to get the nutritional benefits without raising your blood glucose level too much.

Salt

Having diabetes increases your risk of developing high blood pressure and other circulatory conditions, and eating too much salt also increases this risk. If you have been diagnosed with high blood pressure, too much salt can make it worse. Using less or no salt in cooking and not adding salt at the table will help you keep your salt intake within the recommended daily amount of no more than 6g (the equivalent of 2.4g sodium).

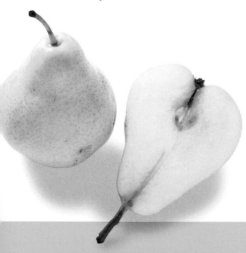

FRESH FRUIT
Fruit is an ideal snack – it is relatively low in calories and full of beneficial vitamins – but eating too much at once means the fructose can raise your blood glucose level.

Practical tips

CUTTING DOWN ON FAT

- Replace butter or full-fat margarines with lower-fat spreads, particularly products that contain monounsaturated fats.
- Use low-fat crème fraîche, greek yoghurt, or low-fat fromage frais instead of full-fat cream.
- Try to eat more fish and poultry – overall these are lower in fat than red meat.
- Choose lean cuts of meat and skinless poultry.
- Avoid fried foods.

Myth or TRUTH?

MYTH
It's okay to eat a small banana, but if you eat a large banana it will raise your blood glucose level.

TRUTH
The days of weighing or measuring foods are over for most people. What matters is the proportion of carbohydrates, proteins, and fats in a meal and the number of portions of fruit and vegetables you eat daily.

Fibre

There are two types of fibre, both of which are important to your health. Insoluble fibre, found in cereals and some vegetables, aids digestion and helps to prevent constipation. Soluble fibre, found in pulses, oats, fruit, and some vegetables, slows down the digestion of carbohydrate and so stops your blood glucose level from rising too quickly after eating. It also helps to reduce your cholesterol level. You should aim to eat around 25g of fibre a day.

Diabetic products and sweeteners

You may come across foods labelled "diabetic" at supermarkets and health food stores. These products are not as beneficial as they sound because they usually contain a sweetener called sorbitol, which is high in calories and makes your blood glucose level rise just as ordinary sugar does. In large quantities, sorbitol will also give you diarrhoea. Diabetic foods are not recommended as they do not help you to control your diabetes – the many low-sugar and low-calorie foods are a much healthier option.

Friends and relatives may buy you diabetic products because they don't know what you can eat and find the labelling reassuring. Let them know that it is fine for you to eat normal chocolate, sweets, biscuits, and similar foods as long as you don't eat them all the time or in large quantities. You can use artificial sweeteners instead of sugar to sweeten food and drinks, such as tea and coffee. These products contain aspartame, saccharin, cyclamate, acesulfame K, or sucralose, none of which affect your blood glucose. However, these products are classed as food additives and have been tested for safety. Because of this, each type of sweetener has a recommended daily amount (shown on the label) that should not be exceeded.

Drinks

Sugary drinks such as glucose drinks, cola, lemonade, and orange juice are digested very quickly, which is why it is recommended that you drink them when your blood glucose level is too low (see pp.106–108). For day-to-day drinks, choose sugar-free substitutes. Tea, coffee, and other hot drinks will not affect your diabetes, but drinking them with skimmed or semi-skimmed milk will cut down on calories. Powdered drinks can have a high

Q **How much alcohol can I drink without affecting my health?**

A The safe limits set by the government's health advisors recommend no more than 3 units of alcohol per day for men, and no more than 2 units per day for women. One unit of alcohol is equivalent to 1 pub measure of spirits, a 125ml glass of wine, or half a pint of ordinary beer. There may be times when you exceed the recommended amounts, however. As with many other things related to your health, an occasional lapse won't do any long-term damage.

ALCOHOL AND BLOOD GLUCOSE

Alcohol contains simple carbohydrate, so drinking will initially raise your blood glucose level – the higher the alcohol content, the greater the effect. In larger quantities, however, alcohol prevents your liver from releasing glucose from its stores, lowering blood glucose and increasing the risk of a hypo occurring.

DRINK	CALORIES	CARBOHYDRATE CONTENT	ALCOHOL CONTENT	EFFECT ON BLOOD GLUCOSE
Pint (568ml) beer	140–185	9–14g	4.5%	Beer causes an initial rise in your blood glucose level. Ordinary bitter has less effect on your blood glucose than strong or real ale.
Pint (568ml) lager	170–230	7.5g	3.2–4%	Lager causes an initial rise in your blood glucose level. Low-carbohydrate/diet lagers will not raise your blood glucose, but can be high in alcohol.
Glass (125ml) dry white wine	80–90	0.7g	9–14.5%	Dry and sweet wines contain similar amounts of alcohol but dry wine has less effect on your blood glucose level because it contains less sugar.
sweet white wine	110–120	7.5g	9–14.5%	
Glass (125ml) red wine	80–90	0.4g	9–14.5%	Red wine contains less carbohydrate than white wine but the effect on your blood glucose level is similar.
Single measure (25ml) spirits	50	trace	40–75%	All spirits have similar amounts of alcohol and calories. On their own they do not greatly raise your blood glucose level.
Glass (25ml) dry sherry	58	trace	15.5–20%	Dry sherries have less effect on your blood glucose than sweet varieties.
sweet sherry	68	3.5g	15.5–20%	

sugar content, so compare labels before you buy. Using artificial sweeteners in drinks instead of sugar won't affect your blood glucose level.

■ **ALCOHOL** There's no reason why you shouldn't drink alcohol when you have diabetes, unless you have been advised not to because of other medical conditions or treatment. However, drinking alcohol initially raises your blood glucose level because it contains simple carbohydrate. In larger amounts it can inhibit your liver's response to hypoglycaemia, which is to release glucose. This increases the risk of a hypo if you take insulin or insulin-stimulating tablets or if you are drinking on an empty stomach. You can reduce the risk of having a hypo by having a meal containing carbohydrate before or while you are drinking alcohol. If you can't eat a meal, snack on sandwiches, crisps, or cereal bars, particularly if you drink more than 2–3 units of alcohol. If you know that you will be drinking a lot of alcohol and food might be in short supply, you may need to take a smaller dose of your tablets or insulin on that day to reduce the risk of a hypo. It is better to have a slightly higher blood glucose level for a short time than suffer a serious hypo that might need hospital treatment.

Practical tips

INCREASING YOUR FIBRE INTAKE

● Add extra fruit to breakfast cereals and yoghurts.

● Have a piece of fruit as a snack instead of a biscuit.

● If you like to snack, keep chopped raw vegetables, such as carrots, celery, and cherry tomatoes, ready prepared in the refrigerator.

● Add beans (such as baked beans) to mince dishes such as shepherd's pie and chilli con carne (this will also reduce the meat and fat content of these dishes).

QUICK AND EASY STIR-FRIES
Stir-frying is an excellent way of cooking vegetables and many other foods. Not only does it require very little oil, but also the cooking time is very short, so food retains its nutritional content.

You should also tell a friend what he or she should do if you have a hypo. People who don't know you might think you are drunk when you are hypo – they won't realize that you need help quickly if your blood glucose level falls too low.

Alcohol is high in calories, so you may need to cut down if you are trying to lose weight or avoid gaining weight. Mixers, such as tonic, cola, and lemonade are high in sugar, so drink low-calorie alternatives to prevent your blood glucose level becoming too high.

Healthier cooking

Having diabetes doesn't mean that you have to forego your favourite recipes. Instead you can adapt your cooking to reduce your overall fat and sugar consumption, include more fruit and vegetables, and generally make sure that your diet is healthy and well-balanced. There are low-fat, low-sugar substitutes for most ingredients in everyday dishes.

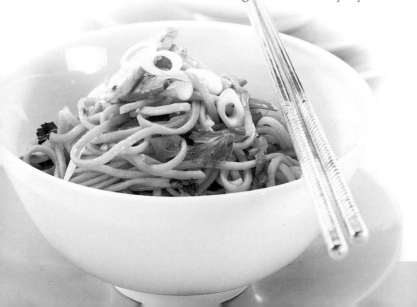

There are also healthier methods of cooking that will reduce calories without compromising flavour.

Recipe adjustment

Try the following ideas for cooking healthier meals:

■ **SOUPS** Use more vegetables to increase fibre and reduce fat content. Avoid adding cream before serving, as the extra fat is unnecessary.

■ **PÂTÉ** Instead of cream and butter or margarine to bind pâté, use a combination of reduced-fat cream cheese and/or half-fat crème fraîche.

■ **CHEESE-BASED STARTERS** To reduce fat content, choose goat's cheese or feta cheese rather than cheese made from cow's milk.

■ **SAVOURY NIBBLES** Lightly brush oil onto spring rolls, filo pastry snacks, or cheese in breadcrumbs and bake them in the oven rather than deep-frying them.

■ **MINCE DISHES** Pre-cook beef or lamb mince to drain off some of the fat. If you are using strong flavourings (spices or curries), try using meat substitutes or soya mince.

■ **PIES** Pastry is high in fat, so use a very thin layer of pastry or make a potato topping instead. Add herbs or chopped spring onions to a mashed potato topping instead of butter.

■ **CASSEROLES** Replace a proportion of the meat or chicken in a recipe with vegetables.

■ **PASTA DISHES** Use tomato-based rather than cream-based sauces.

■ **MAYONNAISE** Use a combination of natural yoghurt and half-fat crème fraîche instead of mayonnaise, which is high in fat.

■ **HOME-MADE ICE CREAM** Use half-fat crème fraîche instead of single or double cream.

■ **TRIFLE** Use plain sponge fingers; fresh, frozen, or tinned fruit (in natural juice); fromage frais instead of cream; and a sprinkle of icing sugar if you need a sweetener. If you are using glazed fruit to decorate, rinse off the preserving sugar.

■ **TIRAMISU** Use virtually fat-free fromage frais and reduced-fat cream cheese in equal quantities instead of eggs and mascarpone cheese. You can still add a small amount of sugar.

■ **CHEESECAKE** Opt for low-fat soft cheese, add fresh fruit, and decorate with grated orange or lemon rind rather than cream.

■ **CRUMBLE** Use porridge oats or wholemeal flour for the crumble to increase the fibre content. Use more fruit filling and less crumble topping.

■ **SPONGE PUDDING** Use half the amount of sugar you normally use to make sponge.

■ **CUSTARD** Use skimmed milk, and add artificial sweeteners instead of sugar after cooking (not before, as this will give the custard a bitter taste).

Cooking methods

Always try to grill, steam, or bake foods rather than fry or cook them in oils or fats. If a recipe requires frying, use cooking oil (see p.36 for healthier types) instead of butter. When cooking meat in the oven, place it on a rack to allow the fat to drain away. Adding herbs also helps to bring out the flavour in food so you can reduce the amount of salt you add to your cooking. You don't have to miss out every high-fat or high-sugar ingredient from a recipe, however, especially if a small amount of that ingredient goes a long way. Parmesan cheese, for example, is high in fat but has a very strong flavour – you would need far more of most other types of cheese to achieve the same taste. Honey, too, may be high in sugar, but a small amount can sweeten a dish more effectively than a large amount of sugar. So if a recipe calls for small amounts of high-fat or high-sugar ingredients, go ahead and use it!

Eating out

There's no need to deny yourself the pleasure of eating out just because of your diabetes. Make healthy choices from the menu – keeping fat and sugar content to a minimum – when possible. If there is no healthy option, don't worry. You can adjust your

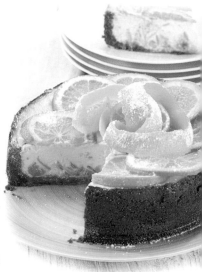

LOW-FAT CHEESECAKE
Reducing the fat content of a recipe doesn't make it any less flavoursome – but it does mean that you can continue to enjoy your favourite desserts as part of a healthy eating plan.

My experience

"It's best to wait until the food arrives before taking your insulin. I've taken insulin when I've ordered, then become hypo because the service is slow. Now I'm on rapid-acting insulin, I can inject just as my meal is being served." SHELLEY

COMMENT Eating out requires a bit of planning ahead because you may not be in control of exactly when you eat. There are different ways of doing this: for example, you could eat lunch a bit later if you are going out for a late dinner, or wait to take your insulin.

Taking a snack with you in case the service is slow will mean you can avoid having a hypo while you are waiting.

medication to accommodate a rise in your blood glucose level if necessary. Even if you don't, the rise will be temporary and your blood glucose level will return to normal once you get back to your usual eating pattern.

The timing of a meal out may be different from your normal eating pattern or you may not be able to predict exactly when you will be eating. This means some forward planning with regard to the timing of your tablets or insulin injections.

You can alter the timing of your tablets or insulin by around two hours without it affecting your overall blood glucose level. If you delay your medication, however, your tablets or insulin may continue working later than normal as a result. Make sure that your tablets or insulin are always timed to coordinate with your intake of food –

it is not a good idea, for example, to take insulin that will work in 15 minutes' time and then not eat for two hours. Taking a snack with you in case the service is slow will mean you can avoid having a hypo while you are waiting.

Choosing from the menu

If you eat out a lot, either socially or because of your work, you will need to pay more attention to the types of food you are eating. An endless round of fast food, pies, rich sauces, or three-course meals will cause your blood glucose level to rise and, in the long term, lead to increases in your weight, cholesterol level, and blood pressure. Although there are times when you don't have any choice, try to follow general healthy eating principles if you eat out regularly.

HEALTHY MENU OPTIONS

Every restaurant menu has options that fit well into a healthy-eating regimen. On the whole, vegetable-based dishes are healthier than meat dishes, but if you want to order meat, one of the "good" options will be lower in fat and calories. You also need to consider what foods accompany your dish, so that your meal is balanced. Ask for advice if you're unsure about ingredients, portion size, or cooking methods.

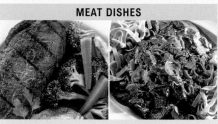

MEAT DISHES

GOOD: STEAK WITHOUT SAUCE

LESS GOOD: BEEF STROGANOFF

GOOD CHOICES: Steak without sauce; roast chicken (with skin removed); grilled lamb steak (with fat removed); stir-fried pork with vegetables.

LESS GOOD CHOICES: Beef stroganoff; steak and kidney pie; steak in creamy sauce; fried lamb chops; burger in a bun.

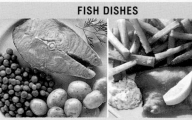

FISH DISHES

GOOD: BAKED SALMON

LESS GOOD: FISH IN BATTER

GOOD CHOICES: Baked or poached salmon or tuna; grilled swordfish steak; smoked mackerel fillets; tuna salad; potato-topped fish pie.

LESS GOOD CHOICES: Fish in batter; deep-fried scampi; fish in creamy sauce; fish in cheese-based sauce.

One way to eat out and stick to a healthy eating plan is to have only two courses for each meal. You can also ask for smaller portions and ensure there is a mixture of foods in your meal. Keep some of the following ideas in mind when choosing from the menu:

■ **STARTERS** Dishes that are deep-fried or drenched in sauce or oil are high in calories and fat. Choose a fruit- or vegetable-based starter instead.

■ **MAIN MEALS** If possible, ask for extra vegetables and a little less meat. Roast, sautéed, and mashed potatoes (which often include butter) are quite high in fat, so opt for baked or boiled potatoes instead. Order sauces in a separate jug so that you can control what goes on your plate.

■ **DESSERTS** Fresh fruit is the healthiest option and is usually available even if it isn't on the menu. If you want to have your favourite pudding, however, ask for a small portion and some fresh fruit to go with it, or share it with a friend. Ask for any cream, custard, or sauce, to be served separately.

■ **DRINKS** Low-calorie or diet drinks are far better for your blood glucose than high-sugar varieties. Fruit juices are also high in sugar.

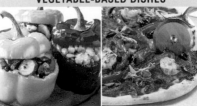

CHANGING TASTES
Seeking out healthier options on the menu can make you more adventurous about food and alter your tastes over time. You may come to prefer lighter dishes with less fat and healthier ingredients.

PASTA DISHES

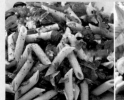

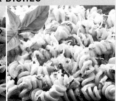

GOOD: PASTA WITH VEGETABLE SAUCE

LESS GOOD: PASTA WITH CREAMY SAUCE

GOOD CHOICES: Pasta with vegetable or tomato sauce; spaghetti Bolognese; pasta with tuna or smoked mackerel; seafood pasta.

LESS GOOD CHOICES: Pasta with creamy sauce, such as carbonara; beef lasagne, pasta with four-cheese sauce.

VEGETABLE-BASED DISHES

GOOD: VEGETABLE-STUFFED PEPPERS

LESS GOOD: VEGETABLE PIZZA

GOOD CHOICES: Vegetable-stuffed peppers; vegetable stir-fry; Spanish omelette; steamed vegetables with rice; ratatouille; grilled vegetable kebabs.

LESS GOOD CHOICES: Vegetable pizza; cauliflower cheese; vegetable samosas; vegetable pasty.

Weight and diabetes

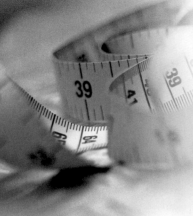

Maintaining a healthy weight is one of the most important steps you can take to manage your diabetes. Being overweight can raise your blood glucose level and cause high blood pressure, increasing your risk of heart and circulatory problems. Where on your body you carry any excess weight is also important. Find out whether you are a healthy weight for your height, why you may lose or gain weight when you have diabetes, and how to lose weight if you need to.

Myth OR TRUTH?

MYTH
You can't lose weight if you have been heavy all your life.

TRUTH
It is possible for anyone to lose weight if they eat less and become more physically active. You need to take one step at a time, use willpower, and set realistic targets to help you to break any habits that you may have picked up over the years. If you find it extremely difficult to lose weight through healthy eating and physical activity, you may be given tablets that will help you.

Why weight matters

Your weight can influence how easy it is to manage your diabetes and can make a difference to the type and dose of any medication you take. Being overweight makes controlling your blood glucose level, blood pressure, and cholesterol more difficult and increases the risk of complications such as heart disease. Keeping your weight within the recommended range for your height (see p.46) or, if you need to, losing a little weight, has many health benefits.

Type 1 diabetes

Rapid weight loss is a common symptom of Type 1 diabetes and a high blood glucose level (hyperglycaemia). Once you start insulin treatment, however, you should put the weight back on. If you have lost a large amount of weight, you will probably need a low dose of insulin to begin with; once

you start to regain weight, you may need to change the dose based on your own day-to-day blood glucose test results. Your weight will also be checked at your annual review and compared with the previous year to assess whether your insulin dose is too high – taking too much insulin may lead to weight gain (see p.46–47).

Type 2 diabetes

You are more likely to develop Type 2 diabetes if you are overweight because being overweight can make your cells resistant to the action of insulin. Four out of five people diagnosed with Type 2 are overweight, so you may well have been advised to lose weight. Even losing a small amount will make it easier to control your blood glucose level, lower blood pressure and cholesterol, and prevent or delay the onset of future complications, such as heart disease.

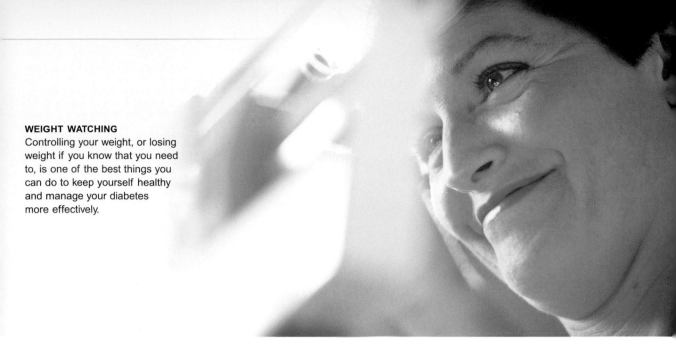

WEIGHT WATCHING
Controlling your weight, or losing weight if you know that you need to, is one of the best things you can do to keep yourself healthy and manage your diabetes more effectively.

You are also likely to need a lower dose of tablets, less insulin, or you may be able to control your diabetes without any medication at all. If you are not overweight, you may want to regain some of the weight you lost or keep your weight within a healthy range.

Why body shape matters

If you carry extra fat around your abdomen rather than around your hips, you have an increased risk of developing heart and circulatory problems. Even if you are overweight, your risk of heart disease is reduced if you have less fat around your abdomen than around your hips. Use the following calculations to assess how your body fat is distributed:

■ **WAIST SIZE** Measure your waist at the widest point. If your waist is more than than 102cm (40in) for a man or 88cm (34in) for a woman, you are carrying too much weight around your middle.

■ **WAIST-TO-HIP RATIO** Measure your waist and your hips at the widest points and divide your waist size by your hip size. For example, if your waist measures 82cm (33in) and your hips 103cm (41in), your waist-to-hip ratio is 0.80. If the result is more than 0.9 (for a man) or more than 0.85 (for a woman) you have a higher risk of developing heart disease.

Is my weight OK?

To assess whether you are overweight you need to measure your body mass index (BMI), which is a ratio of your weight to your height. To work out your BMI, you can either use a chart (see p.46) or calculate it on paper by dividing your weight in kilograms by the square of your height in metres. For example, if you weigh 70kg and your height is 1.67 metres, your BMI is 70 ÷ 2.79 (1.67 x 1.67) = 25. If you have a BMI of 25 or more, you

> If you carry extra fat around your waist rather than around your hips, you have an increased risk of developing heart and circulatory problems.

WORKING OUT YOUR BODY MASS INDEX (BMI)

To find your BMI, measure your unclothed weight and your height. Trace a straight horizontal and vertical line from each measurement on the chart below. The point at which the two lines cross indicates the weight range you are in. You can then decide if you need to gain weight, lose weight, or maintain your healthy weight.

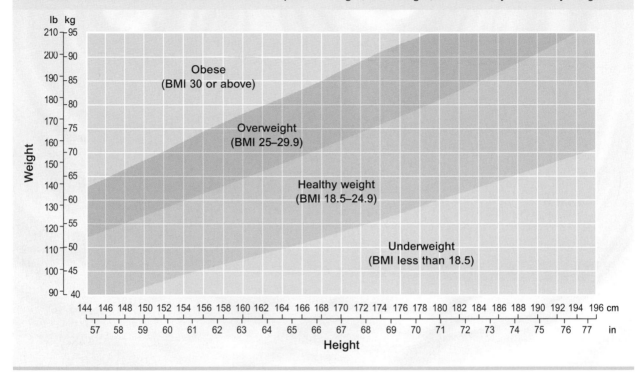

are overweight; if you have a BMI of 30 or above, you are considered to be obese. Obesity carries an even greater risk to your health.

What causes weight loss?

Having diabetes can sometimes make you lose weight unhealthily. The most common reason for weight loss is a high blood glucose level, which means that your body is not using glucose properly for energy. Instead, your body starts to use fat from stores in your muscles and beneath the skin. If your diabetes continues to be uncontrolled, you will start to lose weight. Weight loss is more common and severe at diagnosis in Type 1 diabetes, but can also occur gradually in uncontrolled Type 2 diabetes. You may also lose weight if you have other conditions possibly related to your diabetes that cause weight loss, for example an overactive thyroid.

What causes weight gain?

Some people with diabetes, and particularly those with Type 2, put on weight. There are a number of reasons why you might gain weight:
• Taking more insulin than you need. This is because insulin causes your

body to store glucose as glycogen in your liver and muscles and, if there is a plentiful supply, as fat beneath your skin. You may need to adjust your insulin dose to counter this (see pp.90–95).

• Taking certain tablets to lower your blood glucose level. There are some types that can cause weight gain (see pp.76–81). You may need to consult your health professional.

• Consuming more calories than you need. You might be eating more because you are worried about hypos and want to prevent them, because you are having more snacks to balance with your tablets, or perhaps because you have stopped smoking and are snacking to compensate. Or you may be comfort-eating because you feel low or depressed. You may need to change your eating habits or eat more healthily (see pp.30–43).

• Being less active, perhaps because you are physically unable to take any exercise or because you find it difficult to fit physical activity into your day. You may need to plan how to increase the amount of activity you do (see pp.52–59).

How to lose weight

If you need to lose weight, the best approach – and the way to keep the weight off – is to eat less and be more active. Bringing your weight into the recommended range for your height will be beneficial to your health: your blood glucose level and blood pressure will come down, your cholesterol level will improve, and you will look and feel better.

It is important to lose weight gradually: "quick-fix" diets that lead to rapid weight loss are unhealthy and you are less likely to keep the weight off. You should aim to lose about ½–1kg (1–2lbs) per week. You may find you lose more weight one week than you do the next. This is perfectly normal as your body adjusts to new habits.

You are much more likely to succeed in losing weight if you set yourself practical realistic targets. So the first step towards successful weight loss is to look at what, when, and why you eat so that you can plan what to do differently.

Writing down what and when you eat and drink in a food diary can give you clues as to what unnecessary calories you are taking in and when. It can also show you whether your meals are spread evenly through the day and whether you are snacking unnecessarily between meals. When reviewing your food diary, ask yourself the following questions:

• Do I eat high-fat or high-sugar foods at particular times of the day?

• Do I tend to sample food while I'm cooking?

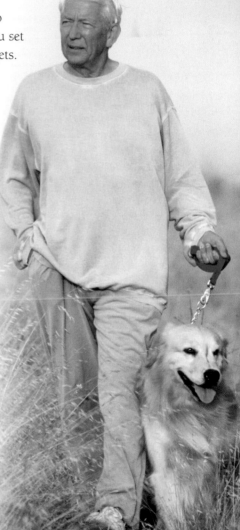

AN ACTIVE LIFESTYLE
Control your weight by keeping active and making sure that you don't consume more calories than your body needs.

Practical tips

MOTIVATING YOURSELF

● Empty your fridge and cupboards of tempting high-calorie foods and replace them with lower-calorie alternatives.

● Keep a record of your successes on a notice board. Don't focus only on your weight – include extra activity and how often you have resisted temptation.

● Put encouraging notes or inspirational pictures on your fridge and cupboard doors to remind you what you are aiming for.

● Ask for the support of a friend or family member you can talk to who will give you encouragement when you need it.

● Do I use ordinary mixers with alcoholic drinks instead of low-calorie or diet versions?
● Do I dine out often and so have less control over what I eat?
● Do I eat very large meals?

If you answered "yes" to any of the above questions, you could make changes straight away to help you lose weight. To keep you motivated on your weight-loss plan, set yourself small targets that you know you can achieve. Aiming to lose 1kg (2.2lbs) by next week, for example, is far easier to work towards than a goal of

losing 20kg (over 3 stone) by next year. Those 1kg (2.2lbs) weeks will soon add up. Even if you only lose half a kilogram (one pound) in a week but are still following your food plan, your weight will continue to fall.

You may also find it useful to set targets related to your food intake rather than your weight. For example, if you decide to cut out or cut down on certain foods during the week, you will feel more positive at the end of the week when you have achieved it – particularly if your weight loss is a little slower than you would like.

USING A FOOD DIARY
Write down everything you eat and drink each day. After a week, review your diary in detail and plan what you could do differently. You could do this with the help of a health professional or friend. Don't forget to congratulate yourself for healthy eating, too!

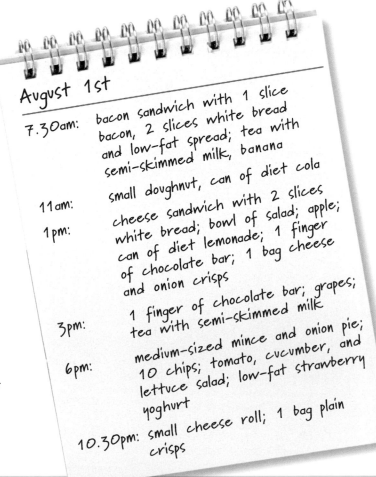

August 1st

7.30am: bacon sandwich with 1 slice bacon, 2 slices white bread and low-fat spread; tea with semi-skimmed milk, banana

11am: small doughnut, can of diet cola

1pm: cheese sandwich with 2 slices white bread; bowl of salad; apple; can of diet lemonade; 1 finger of chocolate bar; 1 bag cheese and onion crisps

3pm: 1 finger of chocolate bar; grapes; tea with semi-skimmed milk

6pm: medium-sized mince and onion pie; 10 chips; tomato, cucumber, and lettuce salad; low-fat strawberry yoghurt

10.30pm: small cheese roll; 1 bag plain crisps

Getting started

"The longest journey starts with a single step". Work through the following questions to help you come up with a plan that will work for you:

- How much weight would you like to lose?
- What specific changes are you going to make to what you eat?
- What specific changes are you going to make to how much physical activity you do?
- How will you change your normal routine to fit in these changes?
- How will you find out how much weight you have lost each week?
- How will you motivate yourself to achieve your weekly targets?
- Who will you ask to help you stay motivated?
- What will you do on the occasions when you aren't able to do what you have decided?
- When will you start your weight-loss plan?

Ask yourself whether what you have planned is realistic. If not, set yourself smaller targets that will bring you greater success. Being successful once in doing what you have planned means you are likely to succeed again.

Once you feel confident that your weight loss plan is achievable, you might find it helpful to take time to list your strategies for overcoming temptation when your resistance is low. Keep the list to hand so that you can refer to it whenever you need inspiration.

My experience

"I cut down my food and insulin, but ate complex carbs so didn't feel hungry. I had hypos at first and adjusted my insulin a lot, but in 8 months I lost 3 stone and needed less insulin overall." SHELLEY

COMMENT When losing weight, you may need to adjust your insulin dose often to avoid hypos or having to eat more to balance your blood glucose. Once you've lost weight, you will need less insulin to control your diabetes.

Calorie counting

The number of calories in food and drink tells you their energy content. To maintain a healthy weight, you need to eat around 2,000 calories per day if you are a woman, and 2,500 calories per day if you are a man.

In order to lose approximately ½kg (1lb) per week simply by eating less, you will need to reduce the number of calories you consume by 500 a day. Fat contains double the calories that carbohydrate provides, so cutting back on fats in your diet is a good start. (See p.36 for the different types of fats and which it

Q Does having diabetes mean that I shouldn't go on a low-carb, high-fat diet – even though it might help me lose weight very quickly?

A Diets that provide extremely different amounts of the main food groups may not be suitable for people with diabetes. A very low carbohydrate intake could cause you to become hypoglycaemic if you take medication for your blood glucose level. If you think a particular eating plan is for you, you should discuss this with your health professional.

You may find it useful to set targets related to your food intake rather than your weight.

can be helpful to cut down on.) However, even if you are eating less, you still need a variety of food types, so excluding an entire type of food, such as carbohydrate or protein, is not healthy. Cutting out carbohydrate is particularly unhealthy as it is your main source of energy, and your body will deplete its own energy stores in its attempt to compensate.

It is better to eat smaller portions of different types of foods instead, making sure that you continue to include all the food groups in every meal and are taking in all of the nutrients you need. Eating fewer than three meals a day is not a good weight loss strategy either – your body needs food at regular intervals to keep your diabetes under control. If you skip meals, you will not only compromise your blood glucose control, but you're also more likely to feel very hungry by the time you do eat, which can lead you to overindulge.

You may need to refer to a book listing the calorie contents of foods and you may have to weigh some foods at first, in order to work out exactly how many calories you are taking in. You can then use your food diary to identify where extra calories are coming from and to decide how to reduce your calorie intake.

You can also look at the labels on packets and tins of food to find out the energy value. Knowing how to read a food label (see left) will help you make healthier choices overall – whether you are shopping for ready-made meals or ingredients for your own cooking.

Some types of food and drink are deceptively fattening, so you may be eating them without realizing how many hidden calories they contain. For example, fruit juice may appear to be healthy, but it is high in sugar; alcohol contains a lot of calories; and some sauces that accompany meals are high in fat.

If you are physically active, you can allow yourself a few more calories and still lose weight. This is because physical activity burns

READING A FOOD LABEL
Compare labels on foods to make healthier choices and assess how much of which ingredients you are eating (ingredients are always listed in decreasing order of weight). If sugar, also called fructose or glucose, is an ingredient, look at its position on the list to gauge the quantity.

Protein Protein is unlikely to cause large fluctuations in your blood glucose level, or affect your weight.

Fat Compare different foods and choose those with a lower fat content (3g or less per 100g) to help you to lose weight. Beware of saturated fats, too, as these can raise your cholesterol level.

Fibre Choose foods with a higher fibre content – fibre not only aids digestion but helps you feel fuller.

Sodium This is the salt content and although it won't affect your weight, limiting your intake (to 0.1g or less per 100g) reduces the risk of high blood pressure.

Carbohydrate The total amount of carbohydrate is given, and also how much of that is made up of sugars. A healthy amount of sugar per 100g is 2g or less – the higher the sugar content, the more chance of weight gain.

Energy Written as kilojoules (kj) and kilocalories (kcals), usually shortened to calories, this is useful if you are calorie counting to lose weight. Generally, opt for low-calorie products.

NUTRITION INFORMATION

Typical values	per 100g	per portion
Energy	1741kJ 414kcal	1219kJ 290kcal
Protein	3.5g	2.5g
Carbohydrate of which sugars	65.8g 49.1g	46.1g 14.4g
Fat of which saturates	15.2g 3.6g	10.6g 2.5g
Fibre	2.3g	2.5g
Sodium	0.1g	0.1g

PER PORTION 290 calories, 10.6g Fat of which 2.5g saturates

calories while you are doing it as well as raising your metabolic rate (the rate at which your body uses up energy) over time. The amount of calories burned depends on the intensity and duration of the activity. (For information on how to increase your activity level, see pp.52–59.)

Dieting and ketones

When you restrict your calorie intake, you force your body to burn its own fat stores for energy, which is why you lose weight. As part of this process, your body may produce toxic by-products known as ketones as it burns fat, which can make your breath smell fruity, rather like the smell of pear drops or of nail varnish remover.

Producing ketones can be normal if you are losing weight, because it is an indication that you are burning fat. You may feel that producing ketones is a good sign because it means that you are being successful in losing weight. However, for people with Type 1 diabetes, producing ketones when you have a high blood glucose level is an indication of a dangerous lack of insulin (see p.113).

EATING BREAKFAST
Don't be tempted to skip breakfast as a way of saving calories – your body needs fuel to start the day. Have a smaller portion and include some fruit if you are trying to lose weight.

CUTTING DOWN ON CALORIES

You can make simple choices on an everyday basis that will cut out calories and help you lose weight without denying yourself the foods you like. Below are some low-calorie alternatives to high-calorie foods and drinks.

HIGHER-CALORIE FOODS	CALS	LOWER-CALORIE FOODS	CALS
100g carbonara sauce	200	100g tomato sauce	70
Small thick-crust pizza	350	Small thin-crust pizza	220
Medium bacon, lettuce, and tomato sandwich	502	Medium salmon and cucumber sandwich	274
300g can cream of tomato soup	216	300g can minestrone soup	93
Chicken breast with skin	300	Skinless chicken breast	190
50g cheddar cheese	215	50g cottage cheese	51
25g blue cheese dressing	115	25g low-fat Italian dressing	22
150g pot greek yoghurt	195	150g pot low-fat yoghurt	80
40g salted peanuts	250	4 bread sticks	84
330ml can ordinary cola	135	330ml can diet cola	0
Small cappucino	70	Regular-sized espresso	4

Physical activity

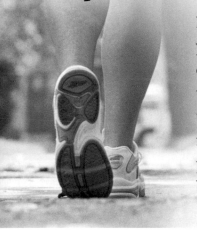

Having a reasonably active lifestyle makes a huge difference to your general health and wellbeing as well as to your diabetes control. Whether you want to walk, dance, or run a marathon is up to you: if you are moderately active on a regular and long-term basis you will feel the benefits. Find out how to get started if you haven't done much physical activity so far, how to devise a plan to meet your individual needs, and how to keep your blood glucose level balanced before, during, and after activity.

Practical tips

FITTING MORE ACTIVITY INTO YOUR DAY

- Walk or cycle short distances instead of driving.
- Get off the bus one stop earlier and walk the rest of the way.
- Use the stairs instead of the lift if you are only going up one or two floors.
- Walk up escalators.
- Incorporate a short walk into your daily routine, perhaps after lunch or in the evening.
- Do some extra gardening or housework.

Being more active

Being physically active is good for you, regardless of whether or not you have diabetes. It strengthens your heart, muscles, and bones, improves circulation, and helps you control your weight. Being active also makes you feel fitter, healthier, and happier, partly because your body is working more efficiently and partly because activity raises your levels of endorphins and serotonin, two brain chemicals that influence your mood and sense of wellbeing. If you are prone to depression (see pp.186–189), physical activity can help to prevent or reduce this.

When you have diabetes, there are even more benefits to be gained from being active – just 30 minutes of moderate activity five times a week can help to regulate your blood glucose level and reduce the risk of long-term complications, such as heart and circulatory conditions.

If you have Type 2 diabetes, regular activity helps reduce insulin resistance, which helps your own insulin to work more efficiently. This may delay the need for increases in dosage of your tablets or mean that you do not need to start taking insulin injections as early. If you have Type 1 diabetes, being more active helps your injected insulin to work more efficiently, so you may be able to reduce your dosage.

How fit are you?

It is a good idea to assess your level of fitness before you start any regular activity. You may be surprised at the amount of activity you already do, or you may feel that you want to do more. Answer the following questions:
- Can you climb one or two flights of stairs without shortness of breath or heaviness or tiredness in your legs?
- Do you normally take the stairs rather than the escalator or lift?

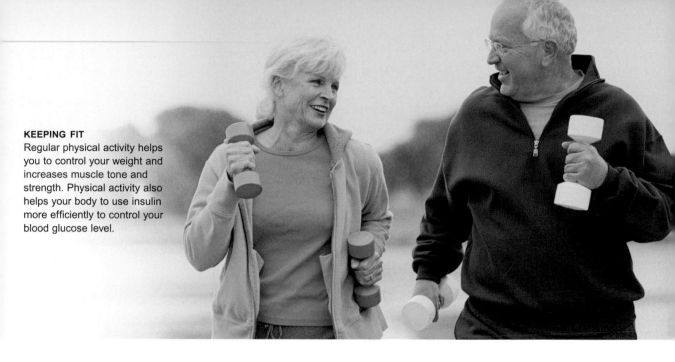

KEEPING FIT
Regular physical activity helps you to control your weight and increases muscle tone and strength. Physical activity also helps your body to use insulin more efficiently to control your blood glucose level.

● Would you walk a 10-minute journey rather than take the car?
● Are you able to carry out a conversation during light to moderate activity, such as walking?
● Do you do 30 minutes of moderate physical activity that makes you sweat and breathe harder at least five times a week?

If you answered "no" to any of the questions above, you could benefit from fitting more activity into your daily routine.

Getting started

Having diabetes places no restrictions on the type of physical activity you can do. If you haven't been active for some time, your best route is to start with any form of gentle activity, assess its effect on your blood glucose level and adjust your diabetes management accordingly. You can then build up your fitness gradually – once your body is used to regular activity you

should aim to be active enough to feel warm and slightly out of breath. If you can sing while you are active, you could probably work harder; if you feel you are gasping for breath, slow down and get your breath back. You should not exercise so hard that you experience any pain.

Physical activity doesn't necessarily mean competitive sports or weight training. It also includes less vigorous pursuits such as walking, gardening,

CALORIES BURNED BY EVERYDAY ACTIVITIES

Day-to-day activities – indoor and outdoor – burn a surprising number of calories. Doing daily chores as part of your activity programme is a good way of boosting your calorie expenditure.

ACTIVITY	CALS PER 30 MINS	ACTIVITY	CALS PER 30 MINS
Climbing stairs	330	Gardening, digging	240
House cleaning	120	Mowing the lawn	140
Shopping	120	Cutting the hedge	120
Ironing	60	Gardening, weeding	105

MOTIVATING YOURSELF

- Set yourself realistic goals and gradually make them more challenging.
- Keep a record of your activity plan and your exercise programme. It can help you to see what you have achieved. It can also help you identify where your plan worked and where it might need to be changed.
- Devise a reward system for yourself to celebrate your success at regular intervals.
- If a situation occurs to prevent you from being active, such as illness or a change in your working hours, don't feel that a lapse means you have failed – revise your plan and get back to your activity as soon as you can.

or housework. Doing something energetic for 30 minutes a day, five times a week, improves your fitness and helps you to control your blood glucose level more easily. You could spread your 30 minutes of activity throughout the day, or work out for an hour three times a week – whichever suits you best.

Building up your fitness

You may find it helpful to work out an activity plan, especially if you haven't been active for some time. The more detailed your plan, the more likely you are to succeed. You may be trying to make long-term changes in your approach to physical activity so it makes sense to look at the big picture right from the start.

Overall fitness is a combination of three factors: stamina, flexibility, and strength. If your aim is to improve your fitness, you need to do regular activity that makes your heart and lungs work harder (to build stamina), improves mobility in your joints (to increase flexibility) and develops your muscle strength.

If you want to lose weight, you may find that gentle activity, combined with changes in your food intake, is enough to achieve this. If not, however, you will need to burn more calories in order to lose weight. You could do this by increasing the intensity of the activity you do, by doing it more often or for longer periods, or by choosing an activity that by its nature burns more calories.

FITNESS BENEFITS OF DIFFERENT ACTIVITIES

When selecting a new activity, you can choose which aspect of your health and fitness to work upon: weight loss, stamina, flexibility, or strength. The fitness benefits of some suggested forms of activity are shown below. One square indicates a small benefit; four squares indicates an excellent benefit.

ACTIVITY	CALS PER 30 MINS	STAMINA	FLEXIBILITY	STRENGTH
Aerobics	215	■■■■	■■■	■■
Cycling (fast)	280	■■■■	■■■	■■■
Golf	195	■	■■	■■
Hiking	200	■■■	■	■■
Jogging	245	■■■■	■■	■■
Swimming (fast)	300	■■■■	■■■■	■■■■
Tennis	210	■■	■■■	■■■
Walking (brisk)	180	■■■■	■■■	■■
Water aerobics	140	■	■■■■	■
Yoga	135	■	■■■■	■

Decide on your goal and then choose an activity that will help you to achieve it. Consider the following to help you determine what you hope to achieve from being more active and how to go about it.

■ **WHY?** Decide what you want to achieve by becoming more active. Do you just want to feel healthier? Would you like to lose weight? Your goal will help you plan which type and how much activity you need to fit into your life.

■ **WHAT?** Think about the type of activity you want to do. If you enjoy it, you're more likely to find the time to do it.

■ **WHEN?** Be realistic about how often you will be able to pursue an activity. Will an activity be part of your normal day (for example walking to the shops), or will you need to find extra time to do it? If you need to find more time, think about when it will be and how you can fit it around your other commitments.

■ **HOW?** Consider what might get in the way of you carrying out your plan. For example, if the time that you set aside for your activity would usually be used to achieve other things, how will you still achieve those things?

■ **WITH WHOM?** Could you team up with a friend, partner, or family member? Teaming up with another person can often make getting fit more enjoyable and give you the support and encouragement you need to stay active.

My experience

"Physical activity is difficult to fit in to my day because I have a young child. But when I make time, I really notice the difference it has on my diabetes control for the next few days." SOPHIE

COMMENT Most people with diabetes find that being active improves blood glucose control. If you are busy, you don't have to take formal exercise. Housework, gardening, and walking can help you to stay active.

Warming up and cooling down

If your chosen activity is fairly intense, it is important to warm up before you begin. You can do this simply by doing your chosen activity at a slow pace for the first ten minutes. This prepares your muscles so that they work better and are less prone

SETTING THE PACE
Regular physical activity improves the flexibility of your joints and minimizes stiffness. To reap these benefits, you need to keep up your activity in the long term, which is why it's important to enjoy whatever you do.

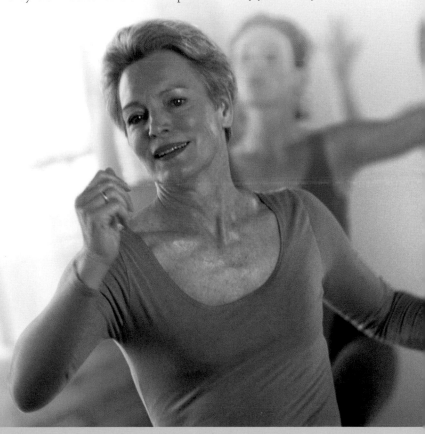

to injury. After your activity, cool down by decreasing the intensity of the exercise for the last ten minutes. Finish by stretching – this is very important to prevent muscle pain and injury.

Managing physical activity and diabetes

When you have diabetes you need to be aware of the effect of physical activity on your blood glucose level and of what action to take to avoid the low and high blood glucose levels it can cause. The effect depends on how intense the type of exercise is (how many calories you burn, see box p.54) and how long you exercise for. If you take insulin or tablets to control your diabetes and you exercise intensively or for a long period, monitoring your blood glucose level particularly closely will help you take action to prevent your activity from causing a hypo.

Physical activity and blood glucose

When you exercise you need extra energy. Your body gets the energy it needs by converting the glycogen stored in your liver and muscles back to glucose. It also gets energy from the fat stored around your body.

Gentle activity for 10–30 minutes is unlikely to have much effect on your blood glucose level. However, if you are more vigorous, your blood glucose level will fall because of the extra glucose your muscles are using. When you stop activity, your muscles and, to a lesser extent, your liver replace their glycogen stores by taking glucose from your bloodstream. The longer or more intense the activity, the more glucose is needed to replenish these stores, so your blood glucose level could be affected for several hours.

Managing blood glucose

Knowing when your blood glucose level is likely to fall will help you identify what – if any – action you need to take. If you are starting physical activity for the first time, test your blood glucose and check the effect that daily physical activities such as shopping and gardening have. If you already do some regular

THE IMPACT OF ACTIVITY ON BLOOD GLUCOSE

If you are moderately active for 30 minutes or more, your blood glucose level changes throughout the activity. The more intense or long-lasting the activity, the greater the impact on blood glucose. Knowing about this helps you decide how to manage your diabetes.

DURATION OF ACTIVITY	EFFECT ON BLOOD GLUCOSE
0–10 minutes	Blood glucose level rises slightly as the body converts glycogen stored in the liver into glucose in the blood.
20–30 minutes	Blood glucose level falls slightly as muscles start to use up available glucose.
30–40 minutes	Blood glucose level could fall even further as more glucose is used up by the muscles to keep them working.
End of activity	Blood glucose level continues to fall as liver and muscles replace their glycogen stores by taking glucose from the bloodstream.

EATING TO CONTROL YOUR BLOOD GLUCOSE LEVEL BEFORE ACTIVITY

Here are some recommendations about whether you should eat – and, if so, examples of appropriate snacks – before you are physically active. Guidelines are based on the intensity and duration of the activity you do, together with your pre-activity blood glucose level in millimoles per litre.

TYPE AND DURATION OF ACTIVITY	BLOOD GLUCOSE BEFORE ACTIVITY	WHAT TO EAT 30 MINUTES BEFORE ACTIVITY
GENTLE: Walking or cycling for less than 30 minutes.	5 or less	1 slice of bread or 1 piece of fruit.
	Any level above 5	Nothing.
MODERATE: Playing golf, leisurely cycling, playing tennis, or swimming for 1 hour.	5 or less	1 slice of bread plus 1 piece of fruit.
	5–9	1 slice of bread plus 1 piece of fruit.
	9–15	Nothing.
	Above 15	Activity not advised until blood glucose level is lower.
INTENSE: Playing football or tennis – for 2 hours. Vigorously cycling or swimming for more than 1 hour.	5 or less	2 slices of bread plus 1 piece of fruit.
	5–9	1 slice of bread plus 1 piece of fruit.
	9–15	1 slice of bread or 1 piece of fruit.
	Above 15	Activity not advised until blood glucose level is lower.

activity, note what effect that has and then compare the effect of more vigorous activity.

If you take tablets or insulin, check your blood glucose level before and after your activity, and again a few hours later. If you are active for more than an hour, it is a good idea to check your blood glucose level in the middle of the activity. If you don't take tablets or insulin, you won't need to make any changes whether your activity is intense or not, although testing your blood glucose might be useful to see what a positive difference physical activity can make.

The following measures will help you keep your blood glucose controlled if necessary:

• If you have a raised blood glucose level before you exercise, and it does not fall as you expect or rises even further, you probably don't have enough insulin to help your muscles use the extra glucose your body is producing. You may need to increase your tablets or insulin dosage to ensure that your blood glucose is well controlled before you exercise.

• If you have Type 1 diabetes and your blood glucose level is over 15 millimoles, avoid exercise until your blood glucose is lower. When your blood glucose level is this high,

Q **Should I avoid physical activity because I have heart problems?**

A Physical activity is particularly important if you already have heart problems, but do consult your health professional before embarking on a fitness regimen. It is important that you start slowly and increase the amount of activity you do gradually over several weeks.

If you are active for more than an hour, it is a good idea to check your blood glucose level in the middle of your activity.

BEING PHYSICALLY ACTIVE SAFELY

● Keep sugary food or drinks available in case your blood glucose level starts to fall while you are active.

● Record your blood glucose level, any changes you make to your tablets or insulin doses, and any extra food you eat to help you to plan for the next time you do similar activity.

● Take your blood glucose monitoring equipment with you if you plan to be active for an hour or more – you may need to do a test.

● Tell someone where you are going and what time you expect to be back if you are planning a long walk, run, or cycle ride.

physical activity may cause it to rise even higher and in this situation ketones may be produced and ketoacidosis (see p.113) may result. Taking your insulin and waiting until it has had an effect will rectify this situation.

● If you know that your activity will make your blood glucose level fall, you could reduce your dosage of tablets or insulin beforehand.

● If your activity is unplanned, or it won't make a big difference to your blood glucose level, you might have an extra snack beforehand rather than adjust your tablets or insulin.

● If you have a low blood glucose level before your activity starts, you will need to eat something – ideally, half an hour before the activity.

● If your blood glucose level is still falling a few hours after activity, you will need to eat something then.

● If you are intensely active for more than an hour, you will need a top up of glucose during the activity – energy drinks or sports bars will give your muscles the extra glucose they need. Energy drinks, every 1–1½ hours will ensure that your body's glucose supplies do not fall too low.

Strenuous activity

If you are active for two hours or more, such as when participating in a marathon or competitive sport, you will need to pay even closer attention to your blood glucose level. If it is too high or low, your performance will be affected and you will tire very quickly. Also, your blood glucose

level might take up to 24 hours to return to normal, as your body replaces the glucose stores in your muscles. Regular testing is essential to monitor your blood glucose level and take action to reduce the chances of having a hypo.

There is no magic formula that will work for everyone, but the following recommendations help keep your blood glucose level steady during strenuous and/or long-lasting activity:

■ **MONITOR YOUR BLOOD GLUCOSE** If you are regularly active for more than an hour, test your blood glucose level before and after activity and also every 1–1½ hours during your activity. You may need to eat or drink something if your blood glucose level is falling. In competitive events, stress and excitement can make you produce hormones, such as cortisol and adrenaline. These hormones can also make your blood glucose level rise – another reason why monitoring is important.

■ **CARRY HIGH-SUGAR SNACKS** Having high-energy food or drink, such as sports bars, bananas, or non-diet

Q Does it make a difference where on my body I inject my insulin before physical activity?

A Yes. If you inject into the limb you will be using, the insulin will enter your circulation much more rapidly. This could cause your blood glucose level to fall too quickly. Choose a different injection site instead. For example, if you are planning a cycle ride, inject your insulin in your buttock or stomach rather than in your leg.

drinks, every 1–1½ hours ensure your body's glucose supplies do not fall too low. Drinking water prevents you becoming dehydrated.

■ **KEEP RECORDS** Knowing the effects of activity and food on your blood glucose level helps you to work out the best way to manage next time.

■ **LOWER YOUR TABLET OR INSULIN DOSE** If you take tablets that help your body produce more insulin (for example, sulphonylureas, see pp.79–80), you may need to reduce the dosage before your activity. Taking a lower dose of your longer-acting insulin the night or morning before the activity, or taking a smaller amount of your shorter-acting insulin with any pre-activity meals, or doing both, will reduce the chances of your having a hypo during your strenuous physical activity.

If you want to increase your muscle bulk or are training for a specific event, such as a marathon, your exercise programme needs to be tailored to your needs. Dealing with endurance sports and diabetes is a specialized subject. You may need advice from your health professional.

Looking after your feet

Most physical activity involves putting extra pressure on your feet. Wear comfortable well-fitting shoes and check that they are appropriate for the type of activity you do. Always check your feet carefully for blisters and other damage before and after activity (see pp.128–130).

ENDURANCE SPORTS
Energy-consuming sports such as marathon running quickly use up glucose in your bloodstream, so you will need to keep topping up with glucose snacks or drinks as you go along.

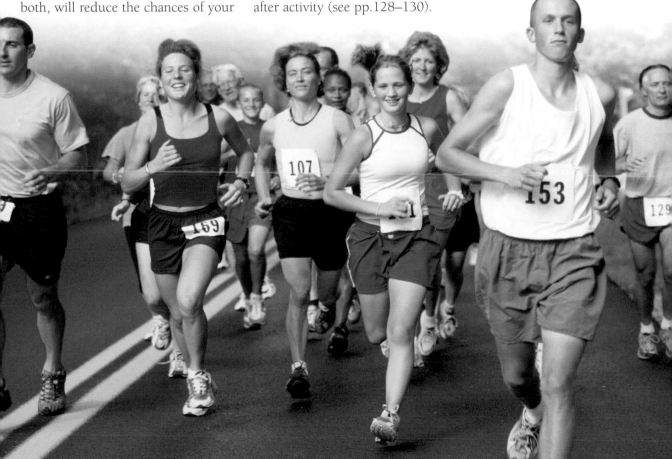

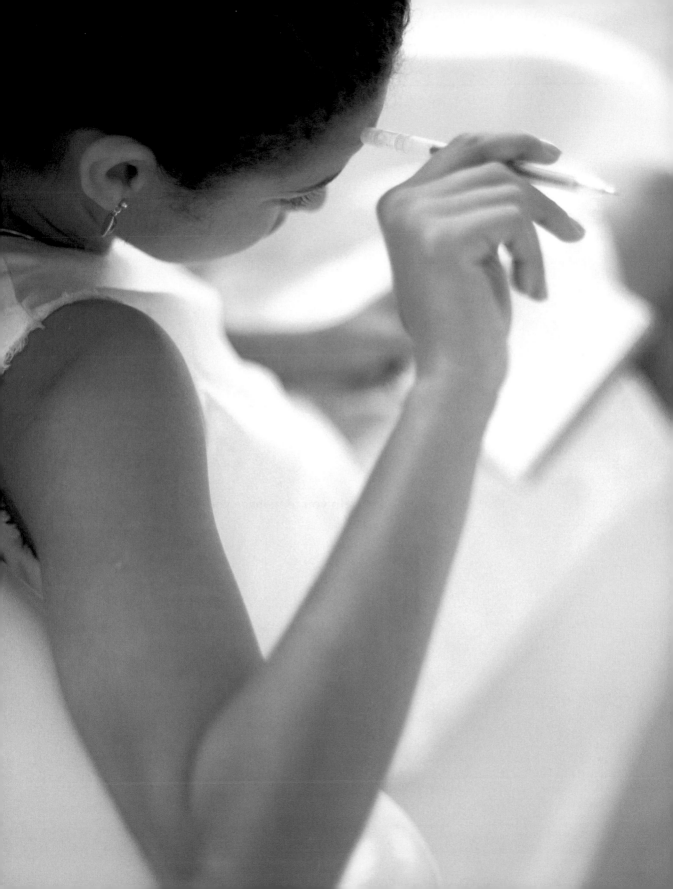

Controlling your blood glucose

By keeping your blood glucose level in the recommended range you feel well and greatly reduce your risk of developing long-term complications.

This chapter gives you the information you need to work towards a blood glucose level that is as well controlled as possible. Frequent blood glucose monitoring and responding to test results accurately will help you to manage your diabetes well.

If you take tablets or other medication for diabetes, it is useful to know how these work and in what combinations they may be prescribed. If you take insulin to control your blood glucose, managing your regimen and learning to adjust your insulin doses when necessary puts you in control of your diabetes.

Even with close attention, instances of low blood glucose (hypoglycaemia) and high blood glucose (hyperglycaemia) are inevitable from time to time. By identifying the causes, however, you can help to prevent them, and by recognizing the symptoms, you can treat them – either yourself or with help.

Monitoring blood glucose

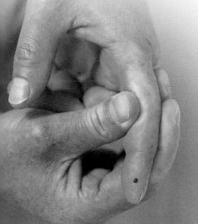

Monitoring the amount of glucose in your blood is part of the daily care of your diabetes. It gives you information about how well you are controlling your blood glucose level, so that you can make adjustments to your treatment if necessary. To manage your blood glucose level in the most effective way, you need to know what level you are aiming for, what causes your glucose level to rise or fall, how to use your monitoring equipment properly, and how to interpret and act on the results.

Understanding blood glucose levels

The goal of treatment for all types of diabetes is to maintain a blood glucose level within a healthy range of 4–9 millimoles of glucose per litre of blood. Although you may experience symptoms if your blood glucose level is lower or higher than this, the only way to know for sure that your blood glucose level is within this healthy range is to take a sample of your blood (or urine; see below) and measure the amount of glucose in it. Regular tests will tell you how your blood glucose level is affected by the food you eat, physical activity, and the medication and/or insulin that you have for your diabetes.

If you start a new kind of diabetes treatment, monitoring your blood glucose gives you vital feedback about how well the treatment is working. Based on the results of your blood glucose tests, you will learn whether the type and dose of a new medication is correct or whether a new or revised regimen of insulin injections is working for you. Alternatively, if you have Type 2 diabetes and you don't yet need medication or insulin, testing can help you to learn about the impact of different foods, drinks, eating patterns, and activities on your blood glucose level.

An HbA1c test (see pp.66–67) is another way of monitoring your

My experience

"Blood glucose monitoring gives me control and helps me understand what's happening in my body. It means I can make the required changes to my insulin amounts accurately." **LOUISE**

COMMENT The information you obtain from testing your blood glucose level means that you are in a position to make immediate adjustments to your insulin. To find out more about making adjustments to your insulin regimen see pp.90–95.

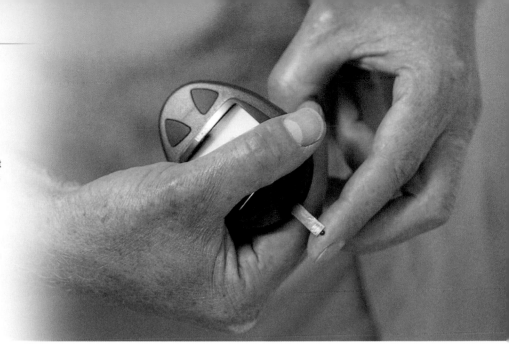

BLOOD GLUCOSE TESTING
To test your blood, you need a blood glucose meter and test strips. If used correctly, meters provide precise and accurate information about your blood glucose level.

blood glucose level. It will generally be performed at your annual review (see p.26) and on one or two other occasions over the course of the year – more frequently if your treatment changes.

Monitoring blood glucose

Testing your blood is the most commonly used method of monitoring your blood glucose level. Other methods are urine testing and continuous glucose monitoring. In the past, urine testing was the standard way to monitor diabetes, but this only tells you when your blood glucose is around 10 millimoles per litre or above. This means you can't exert very tight control over your blood glucose level. However, if you have been taught to monitor your blood glucose by testing your urine, you should not stop doing this without consulting your health professional.

Urine testing is carried out by dipping test strips (these would be prescribed by a medical professional) into your urine and comparing the colour change of the pad with a colour chart.

The procedure for testing your blood is described on pp.70–73 and more information on continuous glucose monitoring is provided on pp.71–72.

How often should I check my blood glucose level?

The general recommendations for useful times to test your blood glucose level are as follows:

- Before each meal – to find out your blood glucose level when it is least affected by food.
- Two hours after each meal – to find out how well your body has used the glucose from your meal.
- Before you go to bed – to find out whether you need to take any action

If you start a new kind of diabetes treatment, monitoring your blood glucose gives you vital feedback about how well the treatment is working.

My experience

"I don't think there is a right or wrong number of times to test per day. I think it should depend on the individual, and how many tests they feel they need to take." SOPHIE

COMMENT What's most important about blood glucose testing is not how many tests you do but how you use the information they provide to make changes to your lifestyle or treatment to keep your diabetes well controlled.

PLANNING A ROUTINE
The number of tests you do each day is up to you, but testing regularly and at standard times can give you a much clearer understanding of what affects your blood glucose level and enable you to identify patterns.

to keep your blood glucose well controlled during the night.

These seven options allow you to build up information about what happens to your blood glucose level at different times of the day (and in response to food). This will help you to identify your usual blood glucose level at these times and give you the opportunity to take action if your blood glucose level is too high or too low. On some days, you may test at all of these times or more; on other days you may do just a few tests or even none at all. The factors that influence how many tests you decide to do each day are as follows:

■ **TYPE OF TREATMENT** You may choose to test at the times when your medication (insulin, tablets, or non-insulin injection) is working at its maximum or minimum effect to ensure that at these times your blood glucose level is not too high or too low. If you do not

take any glucose-lowering medication, you may test at times that measure the effects of different foods, timings, and physical activity.

■ **THE INFORMATION YOU REQUIRE** Sometimes you may choose to test more frequently than usual because you want to find out how your blood glucose responds to a specific situation, such as going for a mile-long walk, eating a particular type of food, or taking a new type of diabetes medication.

■ **GUIDANCE FROM YOUR HEALTH PROFESSIONAL** You may be given specific information by your health professional about how often to test. This is based upon an assessment of how well your diabetes is controlled. Sometimes you might be asked to test more frequently before you attend an appointment with your health professional so that you can both make an accurate appraisal of your blood glucose control.

■ **LEVEL OF CONTROL** If it is very important that you achieve a blood glucose level below 7 millimoles per litre at all times, you need to test frequently to enable you to act on the results. This level of control is necessary in certain situations, such as when you are planning a pregnancy, or if you have early signs of long-term complications.

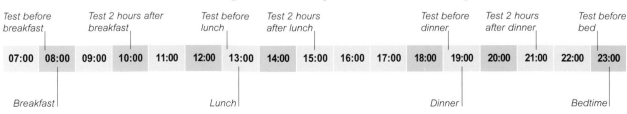

Test before breakfast		Test 2 hours after breakfast			Test before lunch	Test 2 hours after lunch					Test before dinner		Test 2 hours after dinner			Test before bed
07:00	08:00	09:00	10:00	11:00	12:00	13:00	14:00	15:00	16:00	17:00	18:00	19:00	20:00	21:00	22:00	23:00
	Breakfast					Lunch						Dinner				Bedtime

Blood glucose levels to aim for

Blood glucose is measured in units called millimoles and, whatever type of diabetes you have, the recommended blood glucose level to aim for is 4–9 millimoles per litre of blood. This is close to the blood glucose range of a person without diabetes. A blood glucose level in this range keeps you feeling well and helps to protect you from long-term complications. There are occasional exceptions to the 4–9 millimoles per litre recommendation; your health professional can guide you on these. For example, if you have difficulty recognizing hypoglycaemia (see p.106), you may be advised to keep your blood glucose level up to or even above 10 millimoles per litre for a period of time.

When monitoring is especially important

Monitoring your blood glucose is always important, but there are times when you may need to take extra care.

■ **PHYSICAL ACTIVITY** If you are increasing your physical activity or doing a session of vigorous exercise, testing before, during, and up to 36 hours after enables you to act quickly if your blood glucose level falls too low.

■ **CONCEPTION AND PREGNANCY** A high blood glucose level in the few months before conception or during pregnancy can have an adverse effect on your baby's development. Tight blood glucose control, avoiding even occasional

FACTORS THAT AFFECT BLOOD GLUCOSE

These everyday factors have an influence on your blood glucose level. If you understand the effect of each, you can take action to prevent your blood glucose level rising too high or falling too low.

FACTOR	EFFECT
Carbohydrate foods; sugary soft drinks	Raise blood glucose. How quickly and how much depends on the type and quantity.
Physical activity	Lowers blood glucose by helping insulin to work more efficiently and using up energy.
Insulin injections	Lower blood glucose. How quickly and for how long depends on the type of insulin.
Diabetes tablets	Lower blood glucose.
Stress	May raise or lower blood glucose, depending on the circumstances.
Illness	Raises blood glucose.

high levels above 7.8 millimoles per litre, is critical.

■ **LONG-TERM COMPLICATIONS** If you develop the early signs of any long-term complications of diabetes, tight control of your blood glucose level may prevent problems developing further and may help them to improve.

■ **AN UNPREDICTABLE LIFESTYLE** If you have a social life or job in which your routine changes a lot, or if you do shift work, frequent testing tells you what effect this has on your blood glucose level and allows you to adapt the way you look after your diabetes accordingly. Even if your routine changes only for a day or two, it's important to be aware of the effect of this on your blood glucose level.

■ **DRINKING ALCOHOL** Alcohol can cause your blood glucose level to rise initially, then fall; the more alcohol

Myth OR TRUTH?

MYTH
If I test my blood glucose first thing every morning, that tells me how well controlled my diabetes is.

TRUTH
If you do one test a day, you need to vary the times you do it in order to obtain information about your blood glucose level at different times of the day.

ON HOLIDAY
A different routine, climate, and activity level, as well as new foods and eating habits, all affect your blood glucose level.

you drink, the greater the fall. Testing while you are drinking and a few hours afterwards can warn you of possible hypoglycaemia.

■ **ILLNESS** Illness can make your blood glucose level rise very high. Frequent testing, at least every four hours may be necessary to give you the information you need to correct your blood glucose level and prevent you from feeling even more ill. (You may also need to monitor your urine or blood for ketones.)

■ **HOLIDAYS** Your routine may change completely when you are on holiday. Your food and alcohol intake and your levels of activity and stress are all likely to be different from usual. Frequent testing will tell you the impact of these factors on your blood glucose level, so that you can respond.

■ **FREQUENT INSULIN ADJUSTMENT** If you have Type 1 diabetes and you fine tune your insulin doses to your body's requirements, either by injections or using a pump, you need frequent information about your blood glucose level. This enables you to choose an appropriate dose of insulin based on what you are going to eat, or have just eaten, or your blood glucose level at the time. If you manage your diabetes in this way, you may need to test immediately before and two hours after every meal.

The HbA1c test

Apart from testing yourself, there is another important way of gathering information about your blood glucose level: the HbA1c test (each letter is pronounced separately). This is a laboratory test performed by your health professional at your annual review (and usually more often). The test involves analysing a blood sample from your arm or finger. The HbA1c test is not affected by anything that you have recently eaten or drunk. It measures the amount of glucose attached to the haemoglobin in your blood and gives an average picture of your blood glucose level over the previous 6–8 weeks.

If you have an HbA1c test result of 7 per cent or below, this indicates good blood glucose control and is related to a reduced risk of developing long-term complications. A higher result than this, however, may mean that your blood glucose level needs to be more tightly controlled – discussing this with your health professional will help you work out what changes you could make.

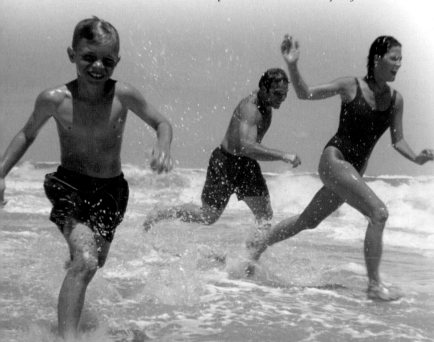

> **Q** **Is it true that my HbA1c test results are going to be given to me differently, and how will I know what the new numbers mean?**
>
> **A** The reporting of HbA1c levels is changing from 1 June 2011, to ensure that HbA1c results are standard throughout the world. The new numbers are in millimoles per mol, rather than a percentage. For example, an HbA1c of 7.0 per cent will be reported as 53 millimoles per mol, or mmol/mol. Until 1 June 2011 you will see your HbA1c result in both measurements, to help you get used to the new values. Your health professional will be able to give you more detailed information.

Monitoring equipment

Specialized equipment is available for you to test your blood glucose level. The most common method of testing is to insert a blood testing strip into a blood glucose meter, then obtain a blood sample using a lancing device, and apply the sample to the testing strip to obtain a reading. Your health professional can help you decide what type of equipment is best for you, or you may obtain information from books, the Internet, or a national diabetes organization (see p.218). You obtain your testing strips and lancets on prescription from your health professional. You can buy meters and fingerpricking devices from a pharmacy or your health professional may give you a starter kit.

Lancing devices

Most lancing devices consist of a hand-held tube, containing a spring, into which you put a needle known as a lancet. A dial on the lancing device enables you to choose the depth to which the needle penetrates (a child would need a shallow setting, such as 1, whereas an adult with thick skin would need a deeper setting, such as 4). Holding the device against the side of your fingertip, you press a button to release the lancet, which pricks your skin. Some lancing devices are designed to take blood samples from areas other than your fingertip, such as your forearm. Lancing devices usually come in a pack with a blood glucose meter, or if not you can contact the individual manufacturer.

Lancets

Small, fine needles, known as lancets, are used with a lancing device to prick

LANCING DEVICES
There is a wide range of lancing devices available, all of which enable you to obtain a blood sample discreetly and with minimum discomfort. You load a lancet into the device, select a depth setting, prime the lancet for action, and press the release button to prick your finger.

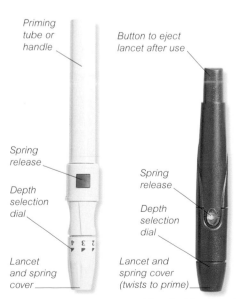
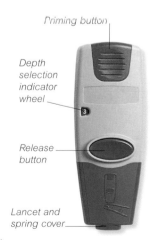

Priming tube or handle

Button to eject lancet after use

Priming button

Depth selection indicator wheel

Spring release

Spring release

Release button

Depth selection dial

Depth selection dial

Lancet and spring cover

Lancet and spring cover (twists to prime)

Lancet and spring cover

Standard lancing devices

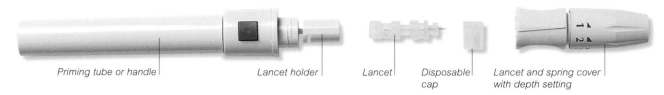

Priming tube or handle   *Lancet holder*   *Lancet*   *Disposable cap*   *Lancet and spring cover with depth setting*

LOADING A LANCET INTO A DEVICE
To insert a lancet into a lancing device you detach the end cover of the device, insert the lancet into the lancet holder, twist off the lancet's protective cap and screw the device together again. The priming handle pulls the lancet back, ready to be released.

Lancets are designed to be used once to avoid infection and also to make sure the needle is as sharp as possible.

your skin and draw a small amount of blood. You insert the lancet into a lancing device, usually by unscrewing part of the device and screwing it together again. Lancets are designed to be used once to avoid infection and also to make sure the needle is as sharp as possible – the sharper the needle, the less pain it causes. Some lancets are universal, which means they fit most lancing devices. Others are specifically made for one type of device. Make sure that the lancets you have are compatible with your lancing device.

Some lancing devices use cartridges that contain a number of lancets, so that you do not have to replace the lancet after every test.

Blood testing strips

Once you have obtained a sample of blood you put it on a blood testing strip. A pack of blood testing strips usually contains 25 or 50. Always check the expiry date of your blood testing strips before use – out-of-date strips do not give an accurate result. Individually packed strips usually last about 2 years. Loose strips in a pot usually last a month after opening (it's useful to make a note of the date when you open a new pot of strips). Most blood testing strips

are designed to be inserted into a blood glucose meter, some are designed to be read visually (see p.73).

Blood glucose meters

Battery-operated devices known as blood glucose meters analyse the amount of glucose in the blood sample on your testing strip and then display the result in millimoles per litre on a small screen. There are two main types of meter: with the most common type, you insert one end of a testing strip into the meter then apply your blood to the other end. The end of the strip inside the meter contains an electrode, which is read electronically by the meter. With the other type of meter, you insert the end of the strip into the meter, then apply blood to the pad of the strip. The meter performs an electronic analysis of the changing colour of the pad.

Both types of meter are highly accurate (provided you follow the manufacturer's instructions) and give results ranging from 0.6–33.3 millimoles per litre.

When choosing a meter, it is worth considering the following features.
■ **SIZE** Some meters are smaller and more compact than others.

If you have arthritis or any other condition that affects your dexterity, you may find a larger meter helpful.

■ **RESULT DISPLAY** Meters with large displays may be easier to read if you have poor eyesight. Some meters give you your test result on its own, others give you the date and time.

■ **MEMORY** Meters vary greatly in the number of results they can store. Some can store 50; others can store up to 500. A large memory is useful if you're often in situations that make it difficult to write down your results.

Q If my blood glucose meter gives me a result in the display screen, can I assume that this is always correct?

A To ensure an accurate result, you must use the meter in the way the manufacturer recommends. If you have not calibrated your meter properly, if you use out-of-date testing strips, or if you do not perform a regular quality control check (see p.71), your meter will not give you an accurate result. Your meter may also give inaccurate results if your blood sample is too small or if it is somehow contaminated – for example, if the site from which you obtain your sample is not clean.

BLOOD GLUCOSE METERS
Blood glucose meters are available in various shapes and sizes to suit individual requirements. Some provide standard functions; others offer additional features or incorporate another device.

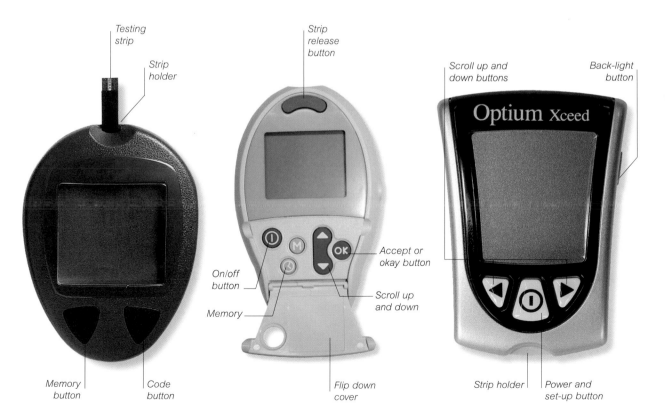

Selection of standard blood glucose meters

Myth OR TRUTH?

MYTH
My blood glucose meter gives me good average readings, so my diabetes must be well controlled.

TRUTH
Unfortunately, average readings can be falsely reassuring. For example, if you frequently have a high blood glucose level in the morning and a low blood glucose level in the afternoon, your average result will disguise these fluctuations. It's worth checking that your average result matches your day-to-day readings.

■ **COMPUTER DOWNLOAD FACILITY** Some meters have a facility that allows you to download your results and analyse them on a computer. This enables you to view your results over a period of time in graph or table form.

■ **AVERAGES** Many meters provide you with an average of your readings, for example over the previous 7, 14, or 28 days.

■ **SIZE OF BLOOD SAMPLE** The amount of blood you need to put on your strip can vary from 0.3 to 4 microlitres. If you find it difficult to obtain blood, it may help to choose a meter that needs a smaller sample.

■ **TIMING** After you have applied your blood, most meters take 5–10 seconds to give you a result. A meter with a shorter analysis time may make it easier for you to test when you are busy.

■ **TESTING SITES** All meters can analyse blood from your fingertips

Q Out of all the meters available, how do I work out which one will suit me best?

A There are no hard and fast rules regarding meter selection. It will largely depend on your personal preference, both for the meter itself and also what features it has that will give you the most useful information to manage your diabetes. Meters vary in size and appearance, and also in how much information they can give you, both immediately and if you download the results onto a computer. Shop around to find out what different meters look like, and the features they have, before making your decision.

but some can also analyse blood from your forearm, the palm of your hand, or your abdomen. If you find your fingers get sore from testing or you use your fingers in your work and taking blood from them is difficult, a choice of testing site can be useful.

■ **ADVANCED FEATURES** Some meters measure both blood glucose and blood ketones (see p.113). Others use a small drum or disc of testing strips so that you don't need to insert a strip every time you test. Ask your health professional for more information about different devices to help you decide whether they would be right for you.

Performing a blood glucose test

It is important that you follow the manufacturer's instructions that come with your testing equipment, to ensure your results are accurate.

Using a blood glucose meter

Depending on the type of meter you have, the exact procedure for carrying out a blood test will vary, which is why it's very important to follow the instructions that come with your meter. However, with most meters, you will need to do the following to obtain an accurate result.

● If you are starting a new packet of strips, you will need to calibrate most types of meter, although some calibrate automatically when the strip is inserted. You may need to carry out a quality control test if you are using the meter for the first time or you haven't done a control test for over a month (see box, below).

• Insert a blood testing strip into your meter – unless the meter contains strips, or you need to apply blood before inserting the strip (your instructions will tell you which).

• Obtain a blood sample (see p.72).

• Apply blood to the testing strip and wait for the meter to display your blood glucose level.

If you insert your strip and then take too long to apply your blood, your meter switches itself off to save battery power. However, once the testing strip has blood on it and is in the meter, an in-built timing device takes over.

Continuous Glucose Monitoring Systems

These systems, known as CGMS, have only become available very recently. Continuous Glucose Monitoring Systems are used when additional information is needed that cannot be provided by conventional blood glucose testing using a meter. They measure the level of glucose in your interstitial fluid, usually in your abdomen, and include:

• A disposable sensor that is inserted into your abdomen and stays in place for up to 3 days.

PREPARING A BLOOD GLUCOSE METER FOR USE

Because blood testing strips vary from batch to batch (they may contain different amounts of chemicals), you need to calibrate most meters every time you start a new pot of strips, to obtain an accurate result. You should also test your meter at least once a month with a quality control solution. The solution contains a known amount of glucose and so enables you to check that your machine is measuring blood glucose correctly.

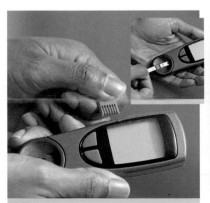

1 If your meter has a coding chip provided with the strips, insert it into the slot on the meter. If it has a coding strip, insert this into the meter, then remove it once the code has been registered. If it has a code (C) button, insert the strip, then press the button until the code matches the new pot of strips.

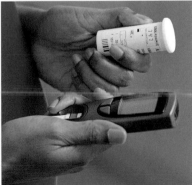

2 When you insert a test strip, compare the code number on the display with the number printed on the test strip pot. The two numbers must be identical. If they are not identical, you need to repeat the procedure until the correct code number is displayed.

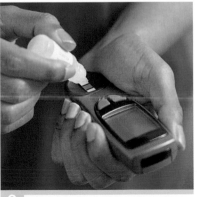

3 To test using the quality control solution, apply the solution to the test strip in the same way as you would apply your blood, then compare the control solution result with the range printed on the test strip or control solution packet. The result should fall within this range.

OBTAINING A BLOOD SAMPLE

The blood test forms part of your day-to-day routine when you have diabetes. Although your finger is the most common site for extracting blood, you can also test blood from your forearm, the palm of your hand, or your abdomen – if your equipment is designed to test blood from these sites. Following these steps will help to ensure that you get an accurate reading from your blood glucose test.

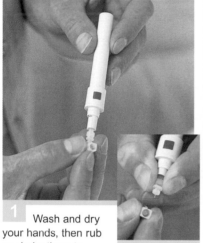

1 Wash and dry your hands, then rub or shake them to maximize your circulation. Make sure you have a fresh lancet available, and remove its disposable cap if necessary.

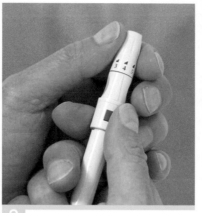

2 Replace the device's cover and turn the dial to set your preferred depth level. Low numbers indicate a shallow depth, higher numbers mean that the lancet goes deeper into the skin.

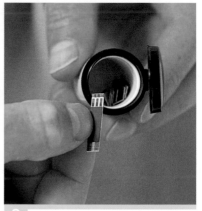

3 Take a fresh blood testing strip out of its packet or pot. Switch on your blood glucose meter or insert the test strip into the meter to switch it on, according to the manufacturer's instructions.

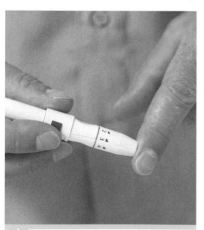

4 Put your lancing device firmly against the side of your finger. Press the button on the side or the end of the device to fire the lancet. Move the lancing device away from your finger and wait a few seconds for the blood to flow.

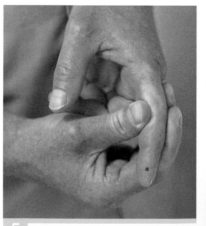

5 If a drop of blood doesn't appear, apply pressure to the base of your finger near the knuckle, moving downwards, to assist blood flow. If you still can't get enough blood, start again using another finger and a new test strip, and increase the depth setting if necessary.

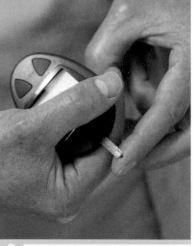

6 When you have enough blood, apply it to the pad on the end of the testing strip. Wait for your meter to display your blood glucose level.

• A rechargeable wireless transmitter that is attached to the sensor.

• A monitor that receives information from the transmitter and displays that information on a small screen.

The sensor measures your glucose level every few seconds and that information is transmitted to your monitor, which gives you an average reading every five minutes. The monitor can also tell you whether your glucose level is rising or falling, and how quickly that is happening. Alarms can be set for high or low readings, and you can also programme your CGMS equipment to alert you a number of minutes before you reach that threshold. This means you can see what is happening to your blood glucose at all times of the day or night, and can find out more about how your blood glucose is affected by your daily activities and food.

There are also CGMS systems which need to be downloaded into a computer before they are analysed. You may be asked to use one of these for a few days by your diabetes health professional, for example to identify specific information about hypoglycaemia. These systems include a sensor, which you wear continuously for up to 3 days and a recorder stores the information about your blood glucose. The recorder is then downloaded so that the results can be analysed.

For all CGMS systems, you still need to carry out some fingerprick blood tests to check the accuracy of the CGMS readings. If you feel you would benefit from using a CGMS device, discuss this with your health professional.

Keeping a monitoring diary

It is important to have a record of your blood glucose tests so that you can see whether your blood glucose level fluctuates over the course of a day or week. You can use a written monitoring diary or, for most meters, you can download your results into a computer. Having a record of the date and time of the test is important, and it is useful to keep a record of any relevant notes, such as what activity you were doing or food you had eaten if you get unexpectedly high or low results. You can also record the time and dose of your medication and/or insulin in a hand-held diary or create a computer log sheet (see p.91).

"I aim for levels of 6–7 millimoles per litre because I am trying to get very tight control. I find I feel hypo if my levels are 5 or below and thirsty if my levels are 9 and above." **SHELLEY**

COMMENT Keeping good control of your diabetes helps you to avoid symptoms on a day-to-day basis. But even if you don't have symptoms, good control is important to prevent health problems in the future.

Practical tips

ENSURING ACCURATE TEST RESULTS FROM YOUR METER

• Read and follow the manufacturer's instructions on how to use your meter.

• Wash and dry the site you intend to take blood from. Dirt or food traces on your skin can produce an incorrect result.

• Each time you start a new pot of test strips, make sure you calibrate your meter and perform a quality control check.

• Always use a new testing strip for each test.

• Don't "top up" blood on your strip if your equipment isn't designed for this. Use another strip and try again.

My experience

"Five tests a day means sore fingers! But it helps me to stay in control of my disease, and have the degree of flexibility that I want in my life." SOPHIE

COMMENT Monitoring is the only way of knowing what your blood glucose level is so that you can take action to keep it controlled. It can mean sore fingers, but it is now possible to obtain blood from other sites, too.

Responding to test results

If you keep your monitoring diary up-to-date, you can examine your blood glucose readings over a period of days or weeks and decide what, if any, action you need to take in response. Rather than focusing on the occasional high or low result, look for patterns. If you have a meter that you can use in conjunction with a computer, you can look at your results in graph or table

USING A MONITORING DIARY
Recording your test results helps you to spot patterns and shows you how different foods, activity levels, and adjustments to your tablets or insulin, if you take them, affect your blood glucose level.

form. Is your blood glucose level always high or low at a particular time of day? The ideal range for your blood glucose level is 4–9 millimoles per litre. If it becomes clear from your monitoring diary that your results are rarely or never in this range, or are constantly swinging between high and low, taking corrective action by, for example, paying more attention to the type or amount of food you eat (see pp.30–43), being more active (see pp.52–59), or changing the dose of your medication (see pp.76–81) or insulin (see pp.90–95) will help to correct this. If these measures don't work or you don't know why your blood glucose level is erratic, contact your health professional even if you are not due for an annual or routine review. You may need a change to your medication and/or insulin regimen.

High blood glucose readings

A single high reading above 9 millimoles per litre with no obvious cause, whatever the level, will happen from time to time and you do not need to take any action. Repeated high readings over a day or more need to be dealt with, however.

The first step is to identify the cause (see box, right) and then act accordingly. So, for example, if your blood glucose level is higher than usual because a muscle strain injury has prevented you

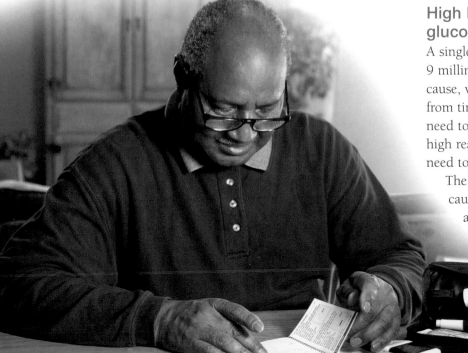

from being as active as usual, you may decide to limit the food you eat or try an alternative activity that doesn't put pressure on the injured muscle.

If stress or illness is causing you to have high readings for a period of longer than one or two days, you can temporarily increase your medication. But remember to return to your usual dose when you are better and your blood glucose level falls. If your weight has increased, you may also need to increase your medication to counteract the insulin resistance this causes.

A high blood glucose level that happens after a hypo, as a result of your hypo treatment and the extra glucose your body produces, can only be prevented by trying to limit the effect of the hypo as much as possible. This may involve reducing your medication or eating more regularly. In all cases, your blood glucose tests will tell you how successful your actions have been (see pp.110–113 for more on hyperglycaemia).

Low blood glucose readings

Blood glucose readings below 4 millimoles per litre should be treated immediately by eating or drinking glucose (see p.106). If you regularly have readings below 4 millimoles per litre, this can reduce your awareness of the signs of hypoglycaemia. A hypo can make it difficult for you to think clearly, but once you are feeling better,

working out the cause will help you plan ahead and prevent it happening again. This might mean reducing your medication, eating more, or altering your activity level.

Whatever course of action you decide to take to prevent a future hypo, your tests will tell you how successful you have been. You may need to make several changes to get the levels you want (see pp. 102–109 for more on hypoglycaemia).

SOME REASONS FOR HIGHS AND LOWS

An occasional high or low blood glucose level does not indicate that your diabetes is out of control (although a low blood glucose level should always be treated promptly). However, if you notice a pattern of highs or lows, finding out why can help you take corrective action.

HIGH READINGS	LOW READINGS
Having more food than usual or a different type of food. (A specific food may be to blame if it's associated with high readings on several occasions).	Having less food than usual, or taking your insulin and/or medication and then being unable to eat at the planned time.
Being less physically active than usual.	Being more physically active than usual.
Illness can cause a high blood glucose reading, as can stress hormones.	Stress can make your blood glucose level fall if you respond to it by using up more energy or eating less than usual.
Forgetting to take your medication or your insulin or taking an insufficient dose.	Taking an extra dose of medication, injecting too much insulin, or being on too high a dose of medication or insulin.
Putting on weight.	Losing weight.
Special circumstances, such as having a hypo earlier in the day, which you treated with glucose (when you are hypo, your liver also converts glycogen into glucose and releases it).	Special circumstances, such as drinking a lot of alcohol without compensating by eating carbohydrate-containing food at the same time or reducing your dosage of medication.

Tablets and other medication

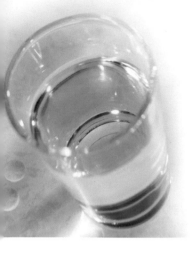

Controlling your blood glucose level with tablets or other medication is likely to be part of your daily routine if you have Type 2 diabetes. No one medication is right for everyone – you may need to try several different types and doses, or take a combination. Whether you are about to start taking medication, or are already doing so, it's useful to know how your particular medication works, information about dosage, and any precautions.

Different medications work better for different people – you may need to try more than one, or different combinations, before you find the one/s that suit you.

Controlling diabetes with medication

Medication is an important way of controlling blood glucose when you have Type 2 diabetes. Although the insulin you produce is insufficient or less effective in Type 2 diabetes, medications used to lower blood glucose levels don't contain insulin, as it would be broken down during digestion. Instead, they control your blood glucose in one or more ways.

- Helping your body to produce more insulin when needed.
- Helping your body cells to use insulin more efficiently.
- Reducing the amount of glucose your liver produces.
- Slowing down your digestion of carbohydrate-rich foods.

Who needs medication?

If you have Type 2 diabetes or MODY (see p.16), you will probably need to start taking medication to control your blood glucose at some point. (If you have Type 1 diabetes, you will always need insulin injections rather than other medication to control your blood glucose.) If, when you are first diagnosed, your blood glucose level is very high (20 millimoles per litre or more) or you have severe symptoms, you will probably be prescribed medication straight away. But, if your blood glucose level is lower than this and you feel well, it is more common for your health professional to recommend that you eat healthily, increase your physical activity, and lose weight if you need to. These measures help to reduce the amount of insulin your body needs, so your own insulin may again be sufficient to effectively control your blood glucose level.

You may be asked to keep your blood glucose level under control in this way for a trial period – usually at least three months – after which your

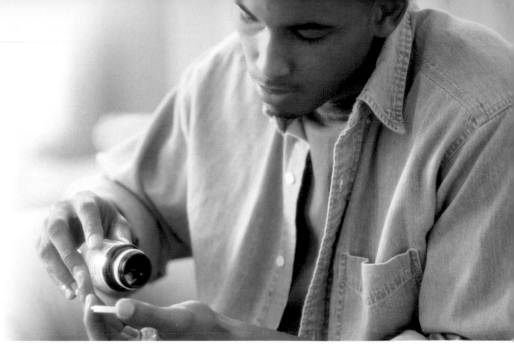

CONTROLLING BLOOD GLUCOSE WITH MEDICATION
Medication prescribed for diabetes works in various ways to lower your blood glucose level. If you have Type 2 diabetes, taking medication, eating healthily, and being physically active are important to keep your diabetes well controlled.

health professional will help you assess how successful this has been. If you need more help to control your diabetes at this or a future assessment, you are prescribed medication. You may manage your diabetes with food, drink, and physical activity for years after diagnosis, or you may need to start taking medication within months.

Being prescribed medication doesn't mean that you have failed to do enough to control your diabetes. It may be because – as is normal in Type 2 diabetes – your pancreas gradually produces less and less insulin over time or your body cells have become increasingly resistant to the action of insulin. It is very likely that you will need medication at some point to control Type 2 diabetes.

The right medication

All medication is prescribed on a trial basis, because it is not until you take it that you discover whether or not it suits you (you may have side effects, for example) and/or is effective. Your health professional is likely to recommend an HbA1c blood test (see pp.66–67) about three months after you have started a new type of medication, to assess how well it is controlling your blood glucose level.

Because Type 2 diabetes is a progressive condition in which your insulin production steadily declines, the dose and type of medication you take need to change accordingly. Your health professional may suggest a gradual increase in the dose of your medication or may prescribe different combinations of medication. More than 30 per cent of people with Type 2 diabetes need to start injecting insulin to control their diabetes at some point. How quickly this happens depends on how long your pancreas can produce enough insulin and how long your medication keeps working to control your blood glucose level.

Myth OR TRUTH?

MYTH
If diabetes medication makes my blood glucose level normal again, I can stop taking them.

TRUTH
Diabetes medication keeps your blood glucose level under control only while you are taking it. If you stop, your blood glucose level rises again. Taking your medication in the right doses and at the right times in relation to food helps to keep your blood glucose controlled in the long term.

These are some of the factors that you and your health professional should consider when choosing the right medication for you.

■ **BLOOD GLUCOSE LEVEL** If the medication you are taking isn't controlling your blood glucose level adequately, you may need an increased dose or one or more different types of medication.

■ **YOUR WEIGHT** If you are overweight, medication that causes weight gain would not be the first choice for you.

■ **THE MEDICATION'S LENGTH OF ACTION** Some medication works over a long period, others only last a short time. Longer-acting medication needs to be taken only once a day, but your chances of hypoglycaemia are higher.

■ **YOUR EATING PATTERN** If your lifestyle means that you don't eat regular meals, medication with a short length of action is more appropriate than longer-acting medication.

■ **SIDE EFFECTS** If you experience side effects, you may need a reduced dose or a different type of medication.

> If your lifestyle means that you don't eat regular meals, medication with a short length of action is more appropriate than longer-acting medication.

Q Can my health professional just keep increasing the dose of my medication each time the medication stops working for me?

A All medications work best when you first start taking them. Increasing the dose after this has some effect on your blood glucose level, but it won't have as much effect as the initial dose. (For example, doubling your dose doesn't have double the effect on your blood glucose level.) This is why your health professional may sometimes prescribe a new type of medication rather than prescribing the maximum dose of your existing medication.

Types of medication

Different medications have different actions, doses, and precautions. Speak to your health professional if you have any concerns about the medication you take. Most medications are not recommended if you are pregnant or breastfeeding. Never exceed the recommended daily dose or stop taking your medication without consulting your health professional first.

Metformin

The first medication you are likely to be prescribed is Metformin (brand name Glucophage) – especially if you are overweight, because it doesn't cause weight gain. Metformin may be prescribed in combination with any of the medications described here.

■ **HOW THE DRUG WORKS** Metformin counteracts insulin resistance by increasing your body cells' sensitivity to insulin. It also reduces the amount of glucose that your liver produces.

■ **DOSE** Metformin comes in combinations of 500mg, 850mg, and 1000mg doses, either as tablets, powder to make into a solution, or slow-release tablets. The dose should start low and increase gradually.

■ **PRECAUTIONS** The main side effects of metformin are nausea and diarrhoea. You can reduce the chances of side effects by always taking Metformin with or after a meal and by increasing doses gradually. For example, if your health professional prescribes four tablets a day, you could build up to this dose by taking one tablet a day for the first week, two a day for the second week, until you are having four a day. You may need to adjust the dose of metformin for some weeks until you discover the amount that controls your blood glucose without producing side effects. If you have side effects on low doses, you may need a different type of medication. Metformin is not recommended if you have kidney problems or severe heart disease.

Sulphonylureas

These medications all work in broadly the same way but have different durations of action, so some need to be taken more times a day than others. The most commonly prescribed sulphonylureas are gliclazide (brand name Diamicron, Diamicron MR), glibenclamide, and glimepiride (brand name Amaryl).

If you are not overweight, a sulphonylurea may be the first type of medication you are prescribed. A sulphonylurea is also commonly added when metformin is no longer controlling your blood glucose level. Other diabetes medications that may be prescribed in combination with sulphonylureas include rosiglitazone, pioglitazone, acarbose, sitagliptin, vildagliptin, and saxagliptin.

■ **HOW THE DRUGS WORK** A sulphonylurea is an insulin-stimulating medication that works on the beta cells in your pancreas to increase the amount of insulin you produce.

■ **DOSE** The dose is a single tablet, which you take just before breakfast.

The dose of shorter-acting sulphonylureas may be increased over time to include more than one tablet per dose and/or a second dose before your evening meal. It is also available as a slow-release medication.

■ **PRECAUTIONS** Common side effects of sulphonylureas include weight gain and hypoglycaemia. Eating regular meals and snacks can reduce the risk of you becoming hypoglycaemic. Your health professional can discuss with you how to adjust your eating if necessary. One sulphonylurea, chlorpropamide, may cause your face to flush when you drink alcohol, and it has a longer action than the other medications in the group, so is more likely to cause hypoglycaemia.

If you have reduced liver or kidney function your health professional may suggest a different type of medication.

Thiazolidinediones

Rosiglitazone (brand name Avandia) and pioglitazone (brand name Actos) are the two tablets in this group. Both tablets are also available combined with Metformin, with the brand names Avandamet (rosiglitazone) and Competact (pioglitazone).

Thiazolidinediones can be prescribed on their own or in combination with metformin or a sulphonylurea, or both, but usually only after you have tried a combination of metformin and a sulphonylurea and this has not been suitable for you. Pioglitazone can also be prescribed in combination with insulin.

Practical tips

REMEMBERING TO TAKE YOUR MEDICATION

● Every morning, count out your medication for the day and check you have taken it all at the end of the day.

● Put the medication in a place that will remind you to take it. For example, by the kettle.

● Prepare your medication at the same time you prepare your meal.

● If necessary, set an alarm for the time you need to take your medication.

● Ask someone to remind you/call you at the time you need to take your medication.

● Always keep a supply of your medication with you so that you can take it wherever you are.

■ HOW THE DRUGS WORK

Thiazolidinediones work by reducing insulin resistance. They also have a beneficial effect on blood pressure, helping protect against cardiovascular conditions (see pp.206–211).

■ **DOSE** Both rosiglitazone and pioglitazone are designed to be taken once or twice a day; either one or two tablets at a time.

■ **PRECAUTIONS** Side effects include weight gain and retaining extra fluid in your body. You should not take thiazolidinediones if you have heart failure or liver problems, or you are taking tablets to get rid of extra fluid in your body. Some thiazolidinediones have, on rare occations, been linked to liver dysfunction so if you take them, you will need your blood tested every few months to monitor your liver function. The risk of bone fractures in women is also increased.

Meglitinides

Repaglinide (brand name Prandin) and nateglinide (brand name Starlix) are faster acting than sulphonylureas and less likely to lead to weight gain and hypoglycaemia. They stimulate insulin production for short periods when you eat and are useful if you have irregular meal times. Newer than sulphonylureas, they are currently less widely prescribed. Repaglinide may be prescribed on its own or in combination with metformin. Nateglinide can be prescribed only in combination with metformin.

■ **HOW THE DRUGS WORK** These medications act on the beta cells in

Side effects of repaglinide and nateglinide include weight gain and hypoglycaemia, but to a lesser degree than other insulin-stimulating medications such as sulphonylureas.

> **Q** Can I adjust my medication dose myself, or do I have to consult my health professional?
>
> **A** Because your need for medication is likely to increase over time, and also because of the importance of controlling your blood glucose level when you are ill, you may need to increase the dosage yourself. If you know how your medication works, for how long, and what the maximum dose is, you can make useful adjustments. Regular blood glucose testing will tell you whether your adjustments have made a difference. It's also important to inform your health professional about changes you've made.

your pancreas to help you produce more insulin.

■ **DOSE** Repaglinide and nateglinide are short-acting, and their effect wears off quickly, so you need to take one tablet before each of your meals. If you miss a meal, you should also miss a tablet, otherwise you risk hypoglycaemia.

■ **PRECAUTIONS** Side effects of these medications include weight gain and hypoglycaemia, but to a lesser degree than other insulin-stimulating tablets like sulphonylureas.

Acarbose

If you already take metformin and an insulin-stimulating tablet (a sulphonylurea, or meglitinide), acarbose (brand name Glucobay) may be added to this combination. It tends to be prescribed less often because side effects are common.

■ **HOW IT WORKS** Acarbose slows the breakdown of carbohydrate during digestion, so that glucose is released more slowly into your bloodstream. Because your blood glucose level then rises more slowly after a meal, your own insulin can cope better.

■ **DOSE** The initial dose is one tablet a day with your evening meal (chewed and swallowed with your first mouthful). The dose should be increased slowly (to avoid side effects), and tablets should be split equally between breakfast, lunch, and your evening meal. The maximum dose is two tablets (200mg) three times a day, but side effects may prevent you from reaching this dose.

■ **PRECAUTIONS** Acarbose can sometimes cause flatulence and diarrhoea. If these are severe, you may need a different type of medication – consult your health professional before you stop taking acarbose.

GLP-1 analogues

Exenatide (brand name Byetta) and Liraglutide (Victoza) are given by subcutaneous injection. They may be prescribed if you are already taking metformin and/or a sulphonylurea but they are no longer controlling your diabetes effectively.

■ **HOW THE DRUG WORKS** Exenatide helps your body produce more insulin when you eat. It also reduces your appetite by slowing down how quickly your stomach empties, so it can help you lose weight.

■ **DOSE** The initial dose of Exenatide is 5mcg twice daily, up to an hour before a meal. This can be increased to a maximum of 10mcg twice daily. For Liraglutide, the initial dose is 0.6mg once a day independently of meals, increasing to a maximum of 1.8mg.

■ **PRECAUTIONS** Exenatide does not cause hypoglycaemia by itself, but it can if taken with a sulphonylurea. If this occurs, the dose of the sulphonylurea should be reduced. Side effects include severe nausea, vomiting, and diarrhoea, which normally wears off after two to three weeks.

DPP-4 inhibitors

Sitagliptin (Januvia), Saxagliptin (Onglyza) and Vildagliptin (Galvus) are DPP-4 inhibitors which help your body produce more insulin when you eat. Vildagliptin is also available combined with Metformin (brand name Eucreas).

■ **HOW THE DRUGS WORK** These medications work by blocking the action of DPP-4, an enzyme that destroys the hormone incretin. Incretins help the body produce more insulin only when needed and reduce the amount of glucose being produced by the liver when it is not needed.

■ **DOSE** The dose of Sitagliptin is 100mg once a day. For Vildagliptin it is 50mg twice a day, unless taken with a sulphonylurea, when the dose is 50mg once a day. For Saxagliptin, the dose is 5mg once a day.

■ **PRECAUTIONS** Common side effects include hypoglycaemia and nausea.

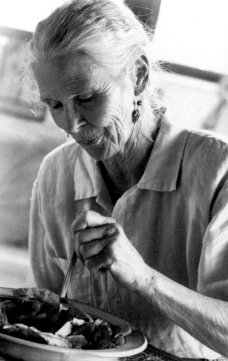

MEDICATION AND MEALTIMES
Taking your medication at the right time in relation to your meal, before, with, or after eating, will help them to be most effective in controlling your blood glucose level.

Insulin

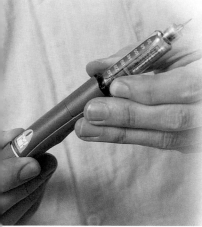

Insulin is essential when you have Type 1 diabetes and is likely to be part of your treatment at some point when you have Type 2 diabetes. There are many types and regimens of insulin and these can be adapted and the doses adjusted to help you get the best control of your diabetes. Knowing about the different delivery devices available – and how to use them – can help you find one to suit you. New forms of insulin delivery may be on the way – alternatives to injections are always being researched.

Controlling diabetes with insulin

Insulin is an essential hormone – without it your body cells cannot take in glucose from your blood to use for energy. This leaves you with little energy and gives rise to other symptoms of diabetes (see pp.18–19). It also forces your body to find alternative sources of energy, such as body fat (see p.113).

If your pancreas no longer produces insulin, or it produces so little that the medication you take for diabetes are no longer effective, you need an external source of insulin, usually in the form of regular injections, although some people receive insulin continuously through a device called an insulin pump. You may be daunted by the idea of injecting insulin, but if you do need it, the many types, doses, and ways of injecting insulin mean that you and your health professional can match your treatment closely to your needs. The aim of insulin treatment is to enable you to feel well on a day-to-day basis and to reduce your risk of long-term complications.

Your insulin regimen (see pp.87–90), will need to change from time to time to ensure that it controls your blood glucose level effectively and matches your lifestyle.

Who needs insulin?

If you have Type 1 diabetes, you don't produce any insulin and your life depends on receiving insulin by injection or insulin pump. If you have Type 2 diabetes or MODY (see p.16), and your blood glucose level reaches the point at which it can no longer be controlled by medication (see pp.76–81), you will also be prescribed insulin. If you have Type 2 diabetes or MODY, you may occasionally need insulin on a temporary basis, for example, if you

Myth OR TRUTH?

MYTH
Human insulin is made from human pancreases.

TRUTH
Human pancreases are not used in the manufacture of human insulin. It is so called because its structure is similar to that of the insulin made naturally in the human body.

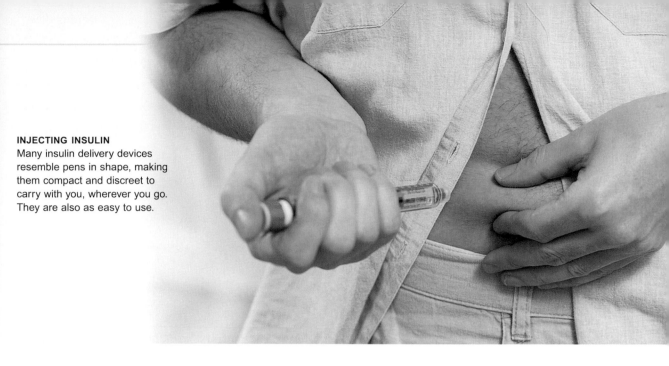

INJECTING INSULIN
Many insulin delivery devices
resemble pens in shape, making
them compact and discreet to
carry with you, wherever you go.
They are also as easy to use.

go into hospital for a major operation,
have a heart attack, or other serious
illness and you are too ill to eat and
drink. In these situations, insulin is
given by infusion (see pp.134–135)
and you may need to continue taking
it by injection after you leave.

If you have gestational diabetes
(see pp.144–145), and changes to
your food intake and activity level do
not control your blood glucose level,
you will need insulin treatment until
the end of your pregnancy, possibly
in addition to other medication. If
you had diabetes that was treated
with other medication before you
became pregnant, you may be able to
continue with it but you are also likely
to need insulin injections.

How insulin controls
blood glucose

The insulin you receive by injection
or pump works in the same way as
the insulin produced in the pancreas
of a person who doesn't have
diabetes. It lowers the level of
glucose in your blood by enabling
your body cells to take in glucose,
and your liver and muscles to store
glucose in the form of glycogen.
Insulin also plays an important part
in preventing glycogen from being
converted back into glucose. This
stops your blood glucose level from
rising unnecessarily. Your insulin
treatment aims to mimic the natural
way insulin is released in your body,
which is to rise and fall according to
the level of glucose in your blood.

Insulin strength and doses

Insulin is measured in International
Units, or "units" for short. There
are 100 units to every millilitre (ml).
Insulin usually comes in either a
small 10ml (1000u) glass bottle,
a 3ml (300u) cartridge, or a 3ml
(300u) delivery device. Unlike
other forms of medication, such as

The insulin
you receive by
injection or
pump works
in the same way
as the insulin
produced in the
pancreas of a
person who
doesn't have
diabetes.

INSULIN PRODUCTION IN A HEALTHY BODY
The pancreas maintains a background level of insulin and produces extra insulin to deal with rises in blood glucose after eating and drinking.

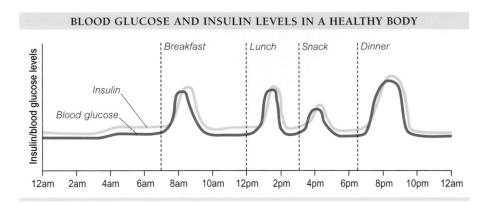

BLOOD GLUCOSE AND INSULIN LEVELS IN A HEALTHY BODY

Insulin/blood glucose levels

Breakfast | Lunch | Snack | Dinner

Insulin

Blood glucose

12am 2am 4am 6am 8am 10am 12pm 2pm 4pm 6pm 8pm 10pm 12am

painkillers or antibiotics, there is no universal maximum dose of insulin. Everyone's needs are different and your insulin dose will be tailored to your needs. You will usually start on a small dose (10–20 units per day) of insulin and increase or decrease this to keep your blood glucose level between 4–9 millimoles per litre. The amount of insulin you need to keep your blood glucose level in the recommended range will vary according to different circumstances (see pp.93–95).

Types of insulin

If you need insulin to control your diabetes, you will be prescribed one or more of four main types. The difference between each type is the length of time it works in your body after you have injected it. You might find that one type of insulin always suits you, or you may need to change types or use different combinations from time to time.

Most insulin used today is "human insulin" which means it has been manufactured in a laboratory to work in a similar way to the insulin produced by a healthy human pancreas. If you have had diabetes for many years, you may take animal insulin, which is produced from the pancreas of a cow or a pig. There are fewer types of animal insulin available than human insulin; it is less commonly used and is no longer likely to be prescribed as a first choice of insulin. However, if you are taking it and you prefer to continue using it, you can still obtain supplies.

Rapid-acting insulin

Rapid-acting insulin is an analogue insulin, which means that it is made by altering the structure of insulin so that it starts working within 5 minutes after you have injected it.

Because it starts working so quickly, you can inject rapid-acting insulin just before you eat or up to 15 minutes after you have eaten. This can be useful when you don't know exactly when your food will arrive or how much of it there will be. Another advantage of taking rapid-acting insulin is that you can make an on-the-spot decision about how much insulin you need in relation to the quantity of food you are eating.

Once rapid-acting insulin is in your bloodstream, it reaches a peak of action after 1–2 hours and wears off after about 4 hours – about the time needed to deal with the rise in blood glucose resulting from your meal. This short duration of action decreases the likelihood of hypoglycaemia between meals.

However, once rapid-acting insulin starts to wear off, your blood glucose level rises. This means that you also need to take a longer-acting insulin – you can mix the two insulins yourself, use a pre-mixed insulin, or take them separately.

Rapid-acting insulin can also be used as a one-off treatment for an unexpectedly high blood glucose level, caused by illness or stress, for example. If you have an insulin pump, you are likely to use rapid-acting insulin. Rapid-acting insulin can be used by both children and adults and there is no evidence to suggest that it shouldn't be used during pregnancy.

Q **Why do shorter-acting insulins tend to be clear and longer-acting insulins tend to be cloudy?**

A Shorter-acting insulins are naturally clear. Most longer-acting insulins are simply shorter-acting insulins that have had protamine and/or zinc added to them to make them last longer. These substances make the insulin appear cloudy. However, insulin glargine and levemir, which are peakless 24-hour-long-acting insulins, are clear.

Short-acting insulin

This is also called soluble insulin and is a clear solution that takes about 30 minutes to start working after you have injected it. For this reason, you need to leave a gap of 20–30 minutes between injecting your insulin and starting to eat. Once short-acting insulin is in your bloodstream, it reaches a peak of action after 2–3 hours and can keep working for up to 8 hours before gradually wearing off.

Because short-acting insulin works for several hours, you may need to balance its action by eating some carbohydrate-containing food as a snack 2–3 hours after a meal – this prevents your blood glucose level

Because short-acting insulin wears off after a relatively short period of time, you also need some longer-acting insulin to ensure you have insulin available through the day and night.

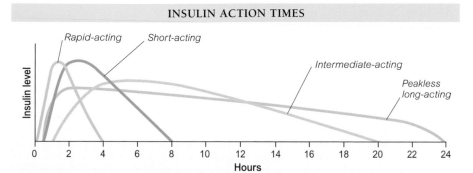

INSULIN ACTION TIMES

Rapid-acting   Short-acting   Intermediate-acting   Peakless long-acting

Insulin level

0   2   4   6   8   10   12   14   16   18   20   22   24
Hours

DURATION OF ACTION
Rapid- and short-acting insulins, start working quickly, and have a relatively short action time – boosting your insulin level to deal with mealtimes. Intermediate- and peakless long-acting insulins have much longer action times, providing a background level of insulin. You may need one type of insulin or more than one type to control your blood glucose level.

falling below 4 millimoles per litre) and making you hypoglycaemic (see pp.102–109). Because short-acting insulin wears off after a relatively short period of time, you also need some longer-acting insulin to ensure you have insulin available through the day and night.

You can mix short-acting and longer-acting insulin yourself or you can use a pre-mixed insulin. You can also take short-acting insulin at mealtimes and a longer-acting insulin at bedtime and/or in the morning.

If your blood glucose level becomes very high, due to illness or stress, for example, you may be taught to correct this by taking an extra dose of short-acting insulin. Short-acting insulin is the type of insulin commonly used in hospital insulin infusions and can be used by people of any age or in any circumstances.

Intermediate-acting insulin

This is also called isophane insulin and is cloudy rather than clear. It is made by adding substances to shorter-acting insulin to make it work for longer – up to about 20 hours. Intermediate-acting insulin reaches a peak of action between 4–8 hours. This helps control your blood glucose level throughout the day, but you may need to eat something around the time of the peak of action to prevent hypoglycaemia. If you have Type 1 diabetes, you may be prescribed an intermediate-acting insulin with a shorter-acting insulin to stop your

---

TESTING THE EFFECT OF DIFFERENT TYPES OF INSULIN

Your health professional prescribes one or more insulins to match your individual medical and practical needs. It's important to understand when different injections of insulin have an effect on your blood glucose level to help you decide when blood glucose tests will be most useful.

TYPE OF INSULIN	WHEN TAKEN	WHEN MOST ACTIVE	WHEN TO TEST BLOOD GLUCOSE
Rapid-acting (Humalog, Novorapid, Apidra) **Short-acting** (Actrapid, Humulin S, Insuman Rapid, Hypurin Neutral)	With or after a meal and 20–30 minutes before a meal	Between that meal and the next meal	2 hours after that meal
Intermediate-acting (Insulatard, Humulin I, Insuman Basal, Hypurin Isophane)	Before breakfast	Between lunch and dinner	Before lunch and dinner
	Before dinner or bedtime	Overnight	Before breakfast
Peakless long-acting (Lantus, Levemir)	At 24-hour intervals	Over a 24-hour period	At any time during the day and night

blood glucose level rising after your shorter-acting insulin has worn off. If you have Type 2 diabetes, you may be prescribed intermediate-acting insulin in this way, or on its own, or with a shorter-acting insulin, or with tablets (see pp.76–81).

Peakless long-acting insulin

This type of insulin, which only became available in recent years, starts working within 30 minutes and is effective for approximately 24 hours. The absence of a peak of action means that you are less likely to experience hypoglycaemia than with other longer-acting insulins.

If you have Type 1 diabetes, you may be prescribed a peakless long-acting insulin in combination with rapid-acting insulin given separately at mealtimes. (You cannot mix peakless long-acting insulin with another insulin in a syringe.) If you have Type 2 diabetes, you may be prescribed peakless long-acting insulin in this way, or on its own, or in combination with other medication.

Insulin regimens

The amount of insulin you need a day and the type or combination of insulin types you use is known as an insulin regimen. Which regimen is best for you depends on the type of diabetes you have and your daily routine.

The regimen prescribed for you when you are diagnosed with Type 1 diabetes or when you start insulin with Type 2 diabetes, is unlikely to be the regimen that works for you permanently. Lifestyle changes such as a new job or a major illness, for example, can significantly alter your insulin needs. Your health professional works with you to decide on the regimen that best controls your diabetes in your particular circumstances.

Once a day

If you have Type 2 diabetes and you need to take insulin as well as other medication, you are likely to start with one injection a day to cover the rise in blood glucose after meals and in the morning. If you have Type 1 diabetes, you would not be prescribed a once-a-day regimen as this would not give you enough insulin to cover your mealtimes.

The insulin prescribed for a once-a-day regimen is an intermediate- or a peakless long-acting insulin. You can inject it at bedtime to avoid morning hyperglycaemia caused by the release of glucose into the blood from the liver during the night. One advantage of bedtime injections is

> The regimen prescribed for you when you are diagnosed with Type 1 diabetes or when you start insulin with Type 2 diabetes, is unlikely to be the regimen that works for you permanently.

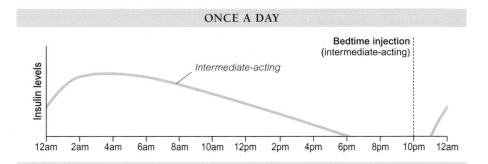

ONCE A DAY

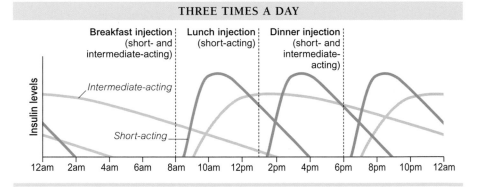

TWICE A DAY

If you have Type 2 diabetes, you may progress from a once-a-day to a twice-a-day regimen if the former does not adequately control your blood glucose level.

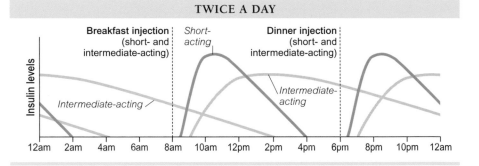

THREE TIMES A DAY

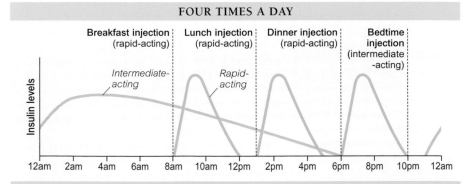

FOUR TIMES A DAY

DIFFERENT INSULIN REGIMENS
These are a selection of insulin combinations for different insulin regimens. Each regimen provides a background level of insulin and the twice-, three-times-, and four-times-a-day regimens give extra boosts of insulin when needed.

that you don't have to remember to carry injecting equipment with you during the day. However, if your lifestyle demands it – if you work night-shifts, for example – you can inject insulin in the morning. Another advantage of a once-a-day regimen is that weight gain and hypoglycaemia are less common than with other regimens.

Twice a day

If you have Type 2 diabetes, you may progress from a once-a-day to a twice-a-day regimen if the former does not adequately control your blood glucose level. You may also be on a twice-a-day-regimen if you have Type 1 diabetes. You may be prescribed one of the following types or combinations of insulin to take twice a day.

• Either an intermediate- or a peakless long-acting insulin.

• An intermediate-acting insulin that comes ready-mixed with a rapid- or short-acting insulin.

• An intermediate-acting insulin that you mix yourself with a rapid- or short-acting insulin.

Whichever of these three options you are prescribed, they are designed so that you inject yourself once in the morning, before or just after breakfast, to control your blood glucose level during the day, and once again in the evening, either before or after your evening meal or before you go to bed, to control your blood glucose level during the night. If your twice-a-day regimen contains rapid- or short-acting insulin, you will need to take it in relation to mealtimes. You need to eat regularly on a twice-a-day regimen to prevent hypoglycaemia.

Three times a day

If you find that a twice-a-day regimen means that there are still times when your blood glucose level is too high, you may be prescribed a third dose of short- or rapid-acting insulin, usually at lunchtime or with your evening meal, depending on the timing of your intermediate-acting insulin.

A three-times-a-day regimen may suit you in the long term or you may only need a third dose of insulin temporarily – for example, if your work or social life has changed recently or you are recovering from an illness.

Four times a day or more (basal-bolus)

This regimen is also known as a multiple injection regimen and it aims to replicate as closely as possible the patterns of insulin rise and falls in a person who does not have diabetes. It is the regimen most likely to be prescribed if you have Type 1 diabetes. You can also use it if you have Type 2 diabetes, you are progressing from a once-a-day regimen and you want a regimen that is more flexible than twice-a-day injections. One or two doses of intermediate- or peakless long-acting insulin in the morning, evening, or bedtime provides a background (known as basal) level of insulin throughout the day. This is supplemented by top-up doses (known as boluses) of short- or rapid-acting insulin either before a meal, in the case of short-acting insulin, or before or up to 15 minutes after a meal for rapid-acting insulin.

A four-times-a-day regimen can help you match the amount of insulin you need to the amount of food you are eating at that time. This helps you to avoid hypos between meals and reduces the number of snacks you need. The longer-acting insulin helps to keep your blood glucose level within a healthy range between the times at which your shorter-acting insulin is working.

Another advantage of the four-times-a-day regimen is that you can make immediate adjustments to your bolus doses based on your activity levels, your food intake, and the results of your blood glucose tests. You can also give extra boluses in certain situations, such as when you are ill or having more meals or snacks than usual.

Continuous delivery

The alternative to single or multiple insulin injections every day is to take insulin continuously by means of a pump (see pp.96–97). You have to wear the pump attached to your body all the time, and you are likely to use a pump if you have Type 1 diabetes and are not able to gain adequate

control of your blood glucose level by more conventional insulin regimens. A pump constantly delivers rapid-acting insulin into your body via a tube in your abdomen. You press buttons to deliver extra doses, called boluses, at mealtimes and when your blood glucose is high. A pump can provide a more flexible lifestyle, mainly because it gives rapid-acting insulin only, so you can quickly adjust your insulin dose to meet your requirements. Using a pump generally requires you to be more active in your diabetes management than other insulin regimens.

Adjusting doses of insulin

An important aspect of diabetes control is adjusting your dose of insulin in response to high or low blood glucose levels, just as the pancreas does if you don't have diabetes. The dose of insulin you need may change when you eat different foods, change your activity level, or are unwell or stressed.

How often you adjust your insulin dose depends on your regimen and your blood glucose levels. You may make frequent adjustments, or you may only adjust your dose in special circumstances, such as holidays or when you are ill. When you start insulin treatment, you are likely to receive frequent advice on dosages from your health professional, but over time, you'll learn to make your own adjustments.

A MONITORING DIARY – USING A FOUR-TIMES-A-DAY REGIMEN

Day	Short-/intermediate-acting insulin injection time and dose				Blood glucose level (millimoles per litre)								Notes/Action
	Breakfast short-acting	Lunch short-acting	Dinner short-acting	Bedtime intermediate	Before breakfast	2 hours after breakfast	Before lunch	2 hours after lunch	Before evening meal	2 hours after evening meal	Before bed	During night	
Mon	6u	6u	10u	20u	7.0	–	14.6	–	10.1	–	6.8	–	BG too high during day. Test again tomorrow.
Tue	6u	6u	10u	20u	7.2	–	14.8	–	9.8	–	6.5	–	Increase morning short-acting by 2 units tomorrow.
Wed	8u	6u	14u	20u	7.5	–	7.2	–	15.3	–	8.2	–	Extra insulin, as out for dinner in the evening.
Thu	8u	6u	10u	20u	7.4	–	7.1	8.6	15.4	–	8.0	–	BG too high before dinner/bedtime. Increase lunchtime short-acting by 2 units.
Fri	8u	8u	10u	20u	8.6	–	7.1	–	12.8	–	6.2	–	Afternoon BG too high – increase lunchtime insulin again.
Sat	8u	10u	10u	22u	8.8	–	7.0	–	7.5	–	6.4	–	Morning BG still too high. Increase evening intermediate.
Sun	8u	10u	10u	22u	3.8	4.6	6.8	–	7.6	–	5.4	–	Hypo this morning; alcohol last night? Reduce bedtime insulin tomorrow if it happens again.

General guidelines

If your home blood glucose tests tend to be outside the healthy range (4–9 millimoles per litre), you need to find out the cause. For example, eating more or less food or being more or less active than usual. You may be able to modify some aspect of your daily routine to bring your blood glucose test results back into a healthy range, but if not, or your changes don't give you the results you need, consider adjusting your insulin dose. Use the following guidelines:

• In general, avoid changing your insulin dose in response to a single test result. Instead, base changes on patterns in your results.
• If your blood glucose level is high for more than a day or two, and other measures aren't working, you need more insulin. Similarly, if your blood glucose level is low for more than a day or two, you need less insulin.
• Start by increasing or decreasing your insulin dose by 2–4 units at

ADJUSTING INSULIN DOSES
Making changes to your insulin in relation to your blood glucose test results is an important part of keeping your diabetes under control. This example shows a regimen of mealtime short- and bedtime intermediate-acting insulin. If you use rapid-acting insulin instead of short-acting, you may make more frequent changes based on the food you are about to, or have just eaten.

Myth OR TRUTH?

MYTH
I have to stay on the insulin regimen I've always had.

TRUTH
There are lots of insulin regimens. The right one for you is the one that keeps your diabetes well controlled but also fits in with your lifestyle. From time to time, you may need to change your regimen to match changes in your daily routine.

a time. If you usually take large doses of insulin, 40–60 units in a single dose, for example, you may need larger dose changes to have an effect – talk to your health professional.

• If you inject insulin more than once a day, change only one insulin dose at a time, so that you can easily check the effect of the change, using your blood glucose test results.

• If you are on a twice-a-day regimen with long-acting insulin, wait at least a day before making further dose changes – this insulin stays in your body for up to 24 hours, so you need this long to assess whether your dose change has worked.

• Children generally need smaller dose changes. For example, 1 unit, or even half a unit, at a time will be effective.

Adjusting a once-a-day dose

You can assess whether your insulin dose needs adjusting by testing your blood glucose level at different times of the day – for example, when you get up in the morning, before or two hours after each meal. If you change your dose and it hasn't brought your blood glucose level under control, consider making a further dose change in a day or two.

Adjusting a twice-a-day dose

If you take intermediate- or peakless long-acting insulin by itself, or intermediate-acting insulin that is ready mixed with a short- or rapid-acting insulin, you need to decide which of your two injections – morning or evening – you need

to adjust. If you want to influence your blood glucose level before lunch, in the afternoon, and before your evening meal, you should adjust the dose of your morning injection of insulin. If you want to influence your blood glucose level in the evening, overnight, and first thing in the morning, you should adjust the dose of your evening injection.

If your changes have not achieved a blood glucose level of 4–9 millimoles per litre, consider making a further change.

Adjusting a three- or four-times-a-day dose

With three- and four-times-a-day regimens, you can make frequent adjustments to your dose of rapid- or short-acting insulin at mealtimes as well as changes to your longer-acting insulin. With rapid-acting insulin in particular, you can inject more or less insulin according to how much carbohydrate is in your meal. If you are not sure how much you are going to eat, you can inject your rapid-acting insulin after you have eaten. You can measure the effect of your dose change by testing your blood glucose two hours later.

If you use short-acting insulin and you change the dose of your breakfast injection, this affects your blood glucose level not just two hours after eating, but up until lunchtime. Similarly, a change in your lunchtime dose continues to affect your blood glucose level in the late afternoon. So an increased dose might cause a hypo 4–6 hours later, even though it corrects a high blood glucose level after 2 hours.

If you notice that your blood glucose level is high or low between meals or first thing in the morning, you may need to change your longer-acting insulin dose. You need to monitor your blood glucose level several times over the day to assess the effect of any change because it is working throughout this period.

Adjusting a continuous dose

If you use an insulin pump, this delivers rapid- or short-acting insulin constantly. Testing your blood glucose every 2–3 hours without eating in between, and assessing how much your blood glucose fluctuates, will tell you if your basal rate is set correctly. If you find it rises or falls more than 1–2 millimoles per litre, you can increase or reduce your dose to prevent this. Your dose adjustments are likely to be much smaller than with injections, possibly only altering your dose by 0.1 or 0.2 units per hour.

For your mealtimes, your insulin dose should match the amount of carbohydrate you eat, and testing your blood glucose before your meal and two hours after will tell you if this is the case. If your blood glucose is more than 2 millimoles per litre from your starting point, you may have miscalculated the amount of carbohydrate you have eaten, there may be other factors (such as a high-fat meal) that have altered the speed of absorption of your meal, or you may need to reassess your insulin to carbohydrate ratio. If your blood glucose level is too high, either two hours after a meal or at any other time, you can give a correction dose based on your usual requirements. You are likely to need to regularly reassess your insulin doses based on your blood glucose readings to get the most out of using your insulin pump.

Dealing with different situations

If you are aware of situations that are likely to significantly raise or lower your blood glucose level, you can take action to prevent this happening.

■ **EATING OUT** If you are going out for a meal or special occasion where you might eat more than usual, you can prevent your blood glucose level rising too high by increasing your dose of insulin before you eat. Alternatively, if you use rapid-acting insulin, you can take insulin after you have eaten and base the dose on the type and size of your meal. When you increase your insulin dose, work

When you increase your insulin dose, work out how long the insulin will stay in your body and when it will have its peak effect.

My experience

"I had to try various regimens before I could control my blood glucose without hypos. This has meant 6 different regimens in 20 years." STUART

COMMENT Adjusting your doses of insulin in response to your blood glucose level can help to keep your diabetes well controlled, but sometimes a change of regimen might give you even more flexibility and control. Your health professional will be able to advise you.

out how long the insulin will stay in your body and when it will have its peak effect (see p.85) – as you may need to have a snack at this point to avoid hypoglycaemia. Also, bear in mind that regularly taking extra insulin to cope with extra food consumption can lead to weight gain. See pp.30–43 for healthy eating guidelines.

■ **PHYSICAL ACTIVITY** Your blood glucose level falls in response to physical activity so, if you are going to be more active than usual, you may need to decrease your insulin dose to avoid hypoglycaemia. For example, if you are going swimming during the morning, you could decrease your morning dose of insulin. Any kind of activity can lower your blood glucose level; dog walking and having sex, for example, are both forms of physical activity.

■ **ILLNESS** A rise in blood glucose is a normal part of your body's response to illness. This happens even if you are not eating and it can slow your recovery time as well as increase the likelihood of diabetic ketoacidosis if you have Type 1 diabetes, and hyperosmolar hyperglycaemic state if you have Type 2 diabetes. For this reason, it is important to increase your insulin dose, based on information from frequent blood glucose tests, to keep your glucose level at least below 10 millimoles per litre. During illness, this increase may be 2–4 units or more at each dose. Alternatively, your health professional may recommend more frequent injections.

As you recover, your blood glucose level usually falls and you will need to reduce your insulin again. Or you may find that your blood glucose level remains high as your body recovers from illness (see pp.130–133).

■ **FASTING** If you are otherwise well and fasting, whether in preparation for a medical investigation or for religious or other reasons, you will need to decrease your insulin dose.

If you have Type 1 diabetes, you need a lower-than-usual dose of insulin for the duration of your fast. If you have Type 2 diabetes, you may be able to have a greatly reduced insulin dose or even stop insulin altogether while you are fasting (because you may still be able to produce some insulin yourself).

If you are not fasting completely but are giving up some types of food, you need to tailor your insulin regimen so that you receive enough insulin when you eat but not so much that

Myth OR TRUTH?

MYTH
When you inject insulin, it goes into a vein.

TRUTH
The insulin you inject yourself doesn't go directly into your bloodstream. Instead, the needle goes into the subcutaneous fat layer (underneath your skin) and the insulin gets absorbed from here into your bloodstream. If you use the correct injection technique, you will not inject into a vein by accident. Sometimes, when you are in hospital you might be attached to an infusion of insulin that goes directly into your vein, but this is temporary and you would never need to do this yourself at home.

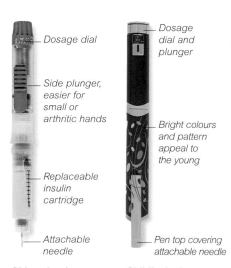

Dosage dial

Side plunger, easier for small or arthritic hands

Replaceable insulin cartridge

Attachable needle

Side-grip plunger device (reusable)

Dosage dial and plunger

Bright colours and pattern appeal to the young

Pen top covering attachable needle

Child's device (reusable)

you become hypoglycaemic at other times. A basal-bolus regimen using a rapid-acting insulin may be useful – ask your health professional.

If you need to fast for a morning medical investigation, you can decrease your insulin dose on the evening prior to the investigation and, if you usually have insulin in the morning, delay this until after the investigation when you are able to eat again.

Insulin equipment

There is a wide variety of equipment designed to deliver insulin. Some people prefer to inject insulin using a needle and syringe; most prefer the convenience of an injection device and insulin cartridge. Receiving insulin continuously via a pump is another alternative. The injection equipment you are offered depends on the type and brand of insulin

Q **What can I do if I am scared of needles?**

A Being scared of injecting before you have ever tried it is common, but true needle phobia is very rare. You may have visions of having to use large needles or inject into a vein. Neither is the case when you are injecting insulin. Try inserting an insulin needle under your skin with your health professional's guidance. You may find this easier and less painful than you expected. This will help to prepare you for giving yourself injections on a daily basis. If you are really phobic, jet injectors, which do not have needles, are available on prescription.

you are taking, as well as your insulin regimen.

■ **INJECTION DEVICES WITH ATTACHABLE NEEDLES** These devices hold 300 units of insulin and consist of a plunger, a dose-dialling system, and an attachable needle. They are a convenient and discreet way to inject insulin. Most devices are pen-shaped and

INSULIN DEVICES
Reusable devices have a replaceable insulin cartridge, or draw insulin from a bottle while disposable devices are ready-filled with insulin. All types use a needle, except for the jet injector, which fires a stream of insulin through the skin under pressure.

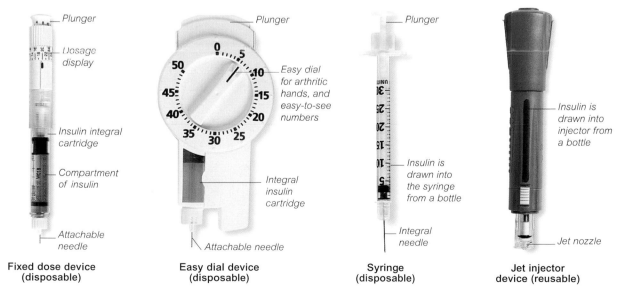

Fixed dose device (disposable)
- Plunger
- Dosage display
- Insulin integral cartridge
- Compartment of insulin
- Attachable needle

Easy dial device (disposable)
- Plunger
- Easy dial for arthritic hands, and easy-to-see numbers
- Integral insulin cartridge
- Attachable needle

Syringe (disposable)
- Plunger
- Insulin is drawn into the syringe from a bottle
- Integral needle

Jet injector device (reusable)
- Insulin is drawn into injector from a bottle
- Jet nozzle

REUSABLE INSULIN DEVICE
Devices such as this one use insulin cartridges, which are inserted into a holder, and have a dose dialling system and a plunger. A new needle is attached each time it is used.

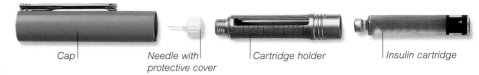

Cap | Needle with protective cover | Cartridge holder | Insulin cartridge

come in either reusable or disposable form. Reusable insulin devices contain cartridges of insulin that you can remove and replace when they are empty. Disposable insulin devices contain an integral insulin cartridge and are thrown away when the insulin runs out – they may last a few days or weeks, depending on how much insulin you take. Whether you have a reusable or diposable device depends on your lifestyle and the brand of insulin you use.

A needle must be fitted to any type of insulin device before use and disposed of afterwards. Needles come in six lengths, ranging from 5mm to 12.7mm. Which length of needle you use depends upon which is most comfortable, and the depth of the fat layer under your skin. The less fat you have, the shorter the needle you will need – children normally require shorter-length needles, for example.

If a needle is too long, you may inject into your muscle, which means that insulin will reach your bloodstream more quickly and cause your blood glucose level to vary unpredictably (see p.98).

■ **SYRINGES WITH NEEDLES** A traditional syringe holds up to 30, 50, or 100 units of insulin and comes with an 8mm- or 12.7mm-long needle already attached. A syringe and needle is smaller than other devices, but you need to draw up your insulin from a bottle each time you inject, so it may be less convenient if you need to inject yourself when you are out.

■ **NEEDLE-FREE JET INJECTOR** This device sends a fine stream of insulin through your skin under pressure, removing the necessity to insert a needle into your body. If you are scared of needles, this device may be of use, although it is larger than most. As with syringes, you need to draw up your insulin from a bottle each time you need a dose.

■ **INSULIN PUMP** A small electronic device that contains a reservoir of rapid-acting insulin. It delivers the insulin constantly through a fine tube, which is connected to a needle or small plastic tube, usually inserted into your abdomen and changed every two or three days. Some pumps have an automatic insertion device to

INSULIN PUMP
An insulin pump delivers insulin continuously through a fine tube into your abdomen via a tiny needle. Pumps can offer good control of blood glucose combined with greater freedom about what and when you eat.

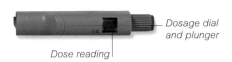

Dose reading — Dosage dial and plunger

put the needle or tube through your skin. An insulin pump keeps a record of what doses of insulin you have received and when. It can be kept inside your pocket or attached to your belt or clothes. Some pumps are waterproof, and you can take off a non-waterproof pump for a short time to bathe or go swimming. If a pump isn't working properly or the insulin is running out, the device will set off an alarm.

Choosing your injection site

Insulin is injected into the fat layer under your skin. The most common injection sites are your thighs, buttocks, or abdomen – your subcutaneous fat layer is too thin

Q **What would happen if I accidentally injected my insulin into a muscle?**

A Insulin would get into your bloodstream more quickly than usual, so you may find that your blood glucose level also falls more quickly. In this situation, you may be more likely to have a hypo. Sometimes, unknowingly injecting into muscle may cause fluctuations in blood glucose. Using a shorter needle or a pinch-up technique (see p.98) can help you to inject insulin correctly into the subcutaneous fat layer.

in other parts of your body. Whichever site you choose to inject into, it is important to change the site frequently. If you repeatedly inject into one site, the frequent exposure to insulin affects your fat cells and causes the area to become lumpy and hard (see lipohypertrophy, pp.212–213).

Although injecting into a lumpy site may be more comfortable than injecting into a non-lumpy site because the skin there has lost sensitivity, this isn't recommended because insulin will enter your bloodstream less efficiently, making it difficult for you to control your blood glucose level. Try to vary injection sites by, for example, injecting into your abdomen for a few days, followed by your thighs and then your buttocks. Even if you prefer to inject one of these sites more than others, make sure that you inject over a wide area within that site rather than restricting all your injections to one small place.

When choosing an injection site, you need to take into account the fact that insulin is absorbed into your bloodstream at slightly different speeds from different sites – fastest from your abdomen and slowest from your buttocks. Insulin also works more quickly if you use the muscles near the injection site vigorously soon after you have injected – for example, if you inject into your thigh and then go cycling. The activity means that insulin circulates much faster than if you injected into a different site.

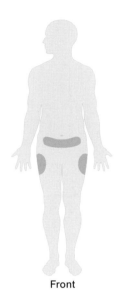

Front

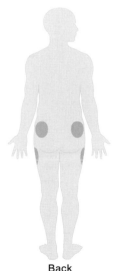

Back

INJECTION SITES
Knowing where on your body to inject your insulin is important. The coloured areas on these diagrams are sites that can be used for injections. You need to change injection sites regularly in order to avoid skin problems.

HOW TO USE AN INSULIN DEVICE

Most insulin devices, whether reusable or disposable, work in the same way, although the details may vary slightly from one device to another – consult the manufacturer's instructions if you are in any doubt. Check the appearance and expiry date of your insulin before you inject yourself (see right). This person is using the pinch-up technique (see right).

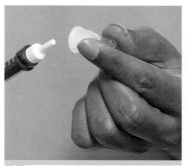

1 Pull off the outer cover of your insulin device and screw a needle into the cartridge in its holder. Remove the needle's inner cap.

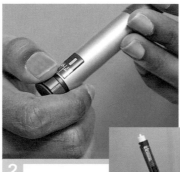

2 If you are injecting a cloudy insulin, rotate your device to ensure it is uniformly cloudy. Dial a small dose of 2–4 units and press the plunger until a drop of insulin appears at the end of the needle (this is called an air shot).

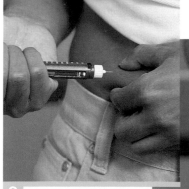

3 Dial the dose that you wish to inject. Then, pinch up a fold of skin at your chosen injection site (in this case the abdomen). Insert the needle into the pinched-up skin, making sure the insulin device is at a 90 degree angle to your body.

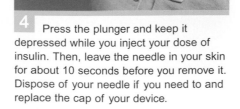

4 Press the plunger and keep it depressed while you inject your dose of insulin. Then, leave the needle in your skin for about 10 seconds before you remove it. Dispose of your needle if you need to and replace the cap of your device.

How to inject yourself

Preparing your insulin and using the correct technique to inject is important in order to enable insulin to work effectively. The precise process of giving yourself an injection depends on whether you are using an insulin device (see box, left), or a syringe (see box, right), but before you inject you need to check your insulin and decide which injection technique you are going to use.

Checking your insulin

Before you inject insulin, check its appearance and expiry date. If it is cloudy when it is meant to be clear, it has a pink tinge, looks lumpy, or contains particles even after gentle rotation, discard it and use a new bottle, cartridge, or disposable device.

Injection techniques

You may have been taught one of two injection techniques.

■ **PINCH-UP TECHNIQUE** This technique involves pinching your skin and subcutaneous fat between your thumb and index finger. Once you have "pinched up", you insert your needle at an angle of 90 degrees. You can release your pinched-up skin when you've finished your injection and removed the needle from your skin.

The pinch-up technique prevents you from accidentally injecting into muscle, but you may not need to use it if you use short needles or if you have a deep layer of subcutaneous fat.

■ **45-DEGREE TECHNIQUE** This involves inserting the needle directly into your skin (without pinching up beforehand) at an angle of 45 degrees. This angle helps to prevent injecting too deeply and reaching the muscle beneath your subcutaneous fat layer if you are using 12.7mm needles.

Insulin and equipment care

The correct way to care for your unopened supply of insulin (whether in bottle, cartridge, or disposable device form) is to store it in a fridge at a temperature of 2–8°C and to discard any insulin that has reached its expiry date (this should appear on the bottle or cartridge, or on the packet of disposable devices). Insulin that is frozen, exposed to high temperatures or direct sunlight, or is out-of-date does not work effectively and should be thrown away.

The insulin that you are using currently (whether in a bottle, reuseable or disposable device) can be safely kept unrefrigerated at room temperature (up to 25°C) for a period of one month. The advantage of this is that, provided you're not in a hot climate, you can carry your insulin around with you without needing to keep it cool. It also means that you don't need to inject cold insulin that has come straight from the fridge (this can be uncomfortable). If you are in a hot climate, you can keep insulin cool by storing it in a cool bag or thermos flask (see p.124).

HOW TO USE A SYRINGE

Check the appearance and expiry date of your insulin before you inject yourself. Discard insulin that is out-of-date or looks different from usual. Ensure that the top of the insulin bottle is clean and use a new syringe each time you inject. This person is using the pinch-up technique (see left).

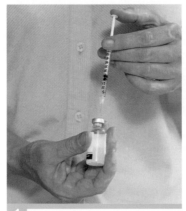

1 For cloudy insulin, rotate the bottle so it is uniformly cloudy. Uncap the needle, draw air into the syringe to match the insulin required. Insert the needle into the bottle and inject the air into the bottle.

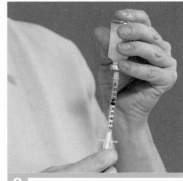

2 Turn the bottle upside down and check that the tip of the needle is in the insulin. Then, pull the plunger back to draw up insulin into the syringe. When you have drawn up the correct dose of insulin, withdraw the needle from the insulin bottle.

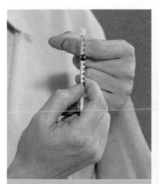

3 Remove any air bubbles by holding the syringe with the needle upwards and flicking the bubbles to the needle end before gently pressing on the plunger to push them out. Check that you still have the correct dose of insulin in the syringe.

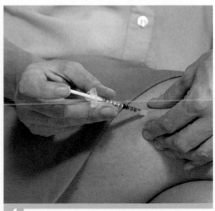

4 Pinch up a fold of skin at your chosen injection site (in this case the thigh) and insert the needle at a 90 degree angle to your body. Press the plunger to deliver the insulin. After injecting, remove the syringe and dispose of it safely (see p.100).

Two recent advances that may offer a realistic way of improving diabetes control and delivering insulin are delivering insulin via inhaler and transplanting islet cells into the pancreas.

Disposing of equipment safely

Syringes with integral needles and attachable needles for insulin devices are designed to be used once only. Reused needles can bend or become blunt, especially if they are very short or fine, and this can make injections uncomfortable. Also, with syringes, the dose markings may wear off with frequent reuse.

When you have finished with a device or syringe and needle, it's important to dispose of it safely to prevent injuries to yourself or others. You can do this by putting the needle or syringe into a puncture-proof container known as a sharps container. Alternatively, you can use a needle-clipping device – after you have clipped the needle from the syringe or device, it is retained in an inaccessible, puncture-proof compartment. A needle-clipping device has the advantage of being small and portable and enables you to use a new needle for each injection when you are out.

Needle-clipping devices can be disposed of in your household waste. Your local council may be able to collect a full sharps container from your home and exchange it for an empty one; or you may be able to collect a new sharps container from your local pharmacy and exchange it when it is full. Ask your health professional about how to dispose of sharps containers in your area. Both sharps containers and needle-clipping devices are available on prescription.

Advances in treatment

From time to time, media headlines highlight research that claims to successfully treat or cure diabetes. This may include transplanting of non-insulin producing cells, which can be altered to enable them to produce insulin, or devices that can automatically deliver the right amount of insulin in response to your changing blood glucose level. Such research is usually in the very early stages, however, and may never fully develop to become a realistic treatment for the majority of people with diabetes. Your health professional will help you identify which treatments are likely to be available to you and also which are likely to be of benefit to you. Transplanting islet cells to enable people to produce insulin again is a treatment option that is now in use. There has also been a wide range of research into trying to find ways of taking insulin without the use of injections, the most promising being inhaled insulin and transdermal insulin.

Islet cell transplant

Transplanting islet cells is a recent advance in treatment that may offer a realistic way of improving diabetes control for a small number of people. If you have Type 1 diabetes, the insulin-producing beta cells, found in the islet cells in your pancreas, have been destroyed. Efforts have been made to overcome this problem by transplanting islet cells or even the whole of the pancreas.

However, transplanting a whole pancreas is a difficult operation and can often be unsuccessful. Islet cell transplants offer a greater chance of success. Islet cells are injected into a vein that leads to the liver, which is a simple procedure that does not require a general anaesthetic. The cells settle in the liver and begin to produce insulin. Most people have been found to need at least two or three transplants of islet cells before they can control their blood glucose level without insulin injections. In some cases, the body's immune system may treat transplanted cells as though they are foreign invaders and attack them. Because of this, islet cells need to be specially treated before they are transplanted. Also, ongoing development of anti-rejection treatment has increased the chances of the cells being accepted by the person's body.

Only a small number of people have so far had islet cell transplants using this technique. However, since February 2008, this treatment has been available at six centres across the UK, having received funding from the Department of Health to provide approximately 80 transplants a year. Exciting as these developments are, and while the treatment will continue to develop and be the subject of important research, it is likely to take many years to become part of routine treatment, so at present, most people who need insulin can expect injections or insulin pumps to continue to be the mainstay of their treatment throughout their lives.

My experience

"The fact that some people have had islet cell transplants gives me great hope. Even if it's not for me, it might help the kids who are being diagnosed today." JOE

COMMENT Islet cell transplants and complete pancreas transplants offer hope that diabetes may be cured in the future, even though it will be many years until treatments like this are available to most people with diabetes.

Inhaled insulin

Many people with asthma take their treatment by inhaler, and the same idea is being applied to insulin. The inhaler would deliver insulin to the lungs as a powder or fine stream of liquid. As with injected insulin, the amount of insulin that is inhaled is critical. Inhaled insulin was introduced in a short-acting format in 2006 and used by a small number of people, but was discontinued in 2008 because at the time it was not economically viable. However, it is likely that at some point in the future, this treatment will be available again.

Transdermal insulin

Another treatment being researched is the use of patches that will slowly infuse insulin when attached to your skin. Progress has been slow as insulin molecules are quite large and that makes it difficult for them to enter your body through your skin. Also, to be successful, the amount of insulin being delivered needs to be very accurate and reliable, and it may mean that people using the patches still need injections of shorter-acting insulin when they eat.

Myth OR TRUTH?

MYTH
An islet cell transplant cures diabetes.

TRUTH
People who have had an islet cell transplant may be able to stop injecting insulin if they produce enough of their own, although they do need to take anti-rejection drugs. Not all people who come off insulin are able to stay off it in the long term.

Hypoglycaemia

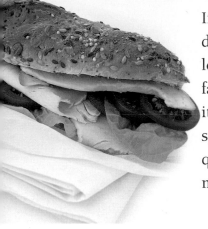

If you take insulin or insulin-stimulating tablets for your diabetes, your blood glucose level may sometimes fall too low – this is known as hypoglycaemia. Being aware of the factors that trigger hypoglycaemia can help you to prevent it happening. If you do have a "hypo", recognizing the symptoms as soon as possible enables you to treat yourself quickly and easily. If your hypo becomes more severe, you may need other people to help you treat it.

What is hypoglycaemia?

Hypoglycaemia – often abbreviated to "hypo" – is the term used to describe a blood glucose level that is too low. In practical terms, this means any level below 4 millimoles per litre, although the level at which you start to experience the symptoms of hypoglycaemia can vary from person to person. Hypos occur when there is more insulin in your body than you need at the time.

If you take insulin, you are certain to have a hypo occasionally. You are also at risk of hypos if you take insulin-stimulating tablets such as sulphonylureas but not if you take other tablets for diabetes, such as metformin, thiazolidinediones, or acarbose on their own (see pp.76–81).

It is important to try to prevent hypos or treat them promptly because a very low blood glucose level can

make you feel unwell, stop you from thinking clearly, make your blood glucose level erratic, and, if it is severe, you may lose consciousness.

The treatment for a hypo consists of eating or drinking glucose, then eating a carbohydrate-containing snack or meal. If you lose consciousness, you will need an injection of glucagon or glucose (see p.109) to raise your blood glucose level. Even after you have treated or been treated for a hypo and your blood glucose level is back within the normal range, you may need some time to recover.

Causes and prevention

Hypos happen when you have too much insulin in your body, perhaps because your insulin or tablet dose doesn't match your food intake or your level of activity or if you have taken, or been advised to take, an

If you have a hypo, it's important to identify the cause so that you can take steps to prevent the same situation from occurring again.

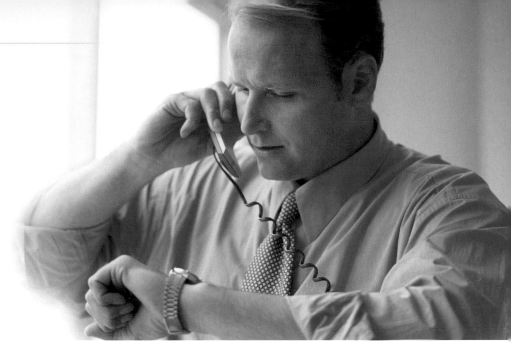

FITTING IN FOOD
A busy lifestyle can sometimes make it difficult to fit regular meals into your day. Missing or delaying eating, however, puts you at risk of hypoglycaemia, so you need to be aware of when to eat, and ensure that you do so, in order to prevent or treat a hypo.

incorrect dose. If you have a hypo, it's important to identify the cause so that you can take steps to prevent the same situation from occurring again.

■ **INSULIN AND TABLET DOSE** If you regularly have hypos, you may need a lower dose of insulin or insulin-stimulating tablets. Dose reductions are commonly needed if you lose weight, you are eating less than usual, you become more physically active, or you have successfully taken a higher dose of insulin to control a high blood glucose level. If you inject yourself with insulin or take insulin-stimulating tablets several times a day, it's important to identify which injection or tablet is responsible if you have a hypo, and then adjust that dose. For example, if your blood glucose level falls before lunch on a few consecutive days, you need to reduce your morning dose of insulin or insulin-stimulating tablets.

■ **FOOD INTAKE** Injected insulin and insulin-stimulating tablets work over a number of hours to control your blood glucose level, and you need to eat during this time to prevent your blood glucose level from falling too low. If you inject insulin, you need to know whether it has a peak of action and, if so, when this is, so that you can balance it with a carbohydrate snack. If you don't balance your insulin dose with carbohydrate-containing food at the right time, you risk having a hypo. Eating later or less than usual, missing a snack, or eating a different type of food, without knowing how much carbohydrate it contains, can increase your risk of having a hypo. If you are unsure about the timing of meals and snacks for your particular insulin regimen, ask your health professional.

■ **ALCOHOL** Although, initially, alcohol causes your blood glucose level to rise, over a period of hours it causes

Practical tips

PREVENTING AND ACTING ON HYPOS

● Check your blood glucose level several hours after vigorous activity.

● If you find it helpful, ask friends, family, or colleagues to remind you to test your blood glucose or to eat snacks at the right times.

● Keep glucose and carbohydrate-containing snacks handy at home, at work, in your car, and on your person.

● If you suspect your blood glucose level is falling, do a blood test to check.

"Like many people who have diabetes I'm frightened of developing complications and I try to reduce my risk by tightly controlling my blood glucose level. I quickly realized, however, that having hypos was the downside of such tight control." STUART

COMMENT Although hypos are more likely when your diabetes is well controlled, they aren't inevitable. One solution is to change to a different type of insulin or tablet. Your health professional will advise you.

your blood glucose level to fall, putting you at risk of a hypo if you take insulin or insulin-stimulating tablets. Hypos when you have been drinking are particularly dangerous because alcohol impairs the corrective mechanism that normally occurs during a hypo, in which the liver's store of glycogen is converted back to glucose and released into the bloodstream. In some situations, hypoglycaemia as a result of alcohol consumption can be life-threatening.

You can prevent this by never drinking alcohol on an empty stomach and, if you drink more than 2–3 units of alcohol, by eating extra carbohydrate-containing food to compensate. This extra food could be crisps, a sandwich, or a take-away meal.

■ **PHYSICAL ACTIVITY** Any sort of physical activity – whether it is housework, shopping, going swimming, or playing a game of tennis – requires energy. Your body's primary source of energy is glucose and the more active you are, the more glucose you burn and the more your blood glucose level falls. You can prevent a hypo in this situation by reducing the dose of your insulin or insulin-stimulating tablets before physical activity or by eating extra food before, during, or after activity.

Long-lasting or strenuous activity requires more careful planning (see pp.58–59). Remember that staying active helps all your body systems to work more efficiently and is important for your long-term health – and with some careful preparations you can prevent your blood glucose level from falling (see pp.56–58).

■ **STRESS** Stress usually makes your blood glucose level rise because the stress hormones adrenaline and cortisol not only oppose the action of insulin, but also cause glycogen in your liver to be converted into glucose and released into your bloodstream. However, stress can also cause your blood glucose level to fall because your body may use extra energy when you are stressed or you may not eat regularly. Try to establish what effect stress has on your blood glucose level. If you know that it lowers your blood glucose level, you can deal with stressful situations by eating extra food or reducing the dose of your insulin or insulin-stimulating tablets.

■ **HEAT** Exposure to heat causes your blood to circulate more quickly, which means that insulin and insulin-stimulating tablets work faster than usual. This in turn causes your blood glucose level to fall. You may find that you are prone to hypos in hot weather.

Checking your blood glucose before taking a hot bath, sauna, or using a sunbed will help you identify if you are close to a hypo and whether you need extra food to avoid this. In future similar situations, you may need to reduce your dose of insulin or insulin-stimulating tablets or eat extra food before or after these activities.

Symptoms

The symptoms of a hypo fall into two categories: early warning symptoms, when your blood glucose level starts to drop, and later symptoms, when your blood glucose level is so low that your brain is not receiving sufficient glucose. The symptoms are more pronounced for some people than for others. If you can't detect and treat your own symptoms, you may need to rely on people around you for help.

Early warning symptoms

You may have any of the following symptoms when your blood glucose level starts to fall:
- Sweating.
- Trembling.
- Feeling anxious.
- Turning pale.
- Palpitations.
- Feeling hungry.

   You may not have all or even any of these symptoms; it's also possible to experience these symptoms in response to any fall in blood glucose – for example, a fall from 15 millimoles per litre to 10 millimoles per litre. Testing your blood glucose

level will give you the information you need to decide whether any action is necessary. Bear in mind, though, that a blood glucose test result does not reveal how quickly your blood glucose level is changing – if you have symptoms and your test result is 4 millimoles per litre, you should treat yourself for hypoglycaemia immediately rather than waiting for your blood glucose level to fall further.

Later symptoms

As your blood glucose level falls below 3 millimoles per litre, your brain is no longer receiving a sufficient amount of glucose. This means that although you may know that you are having a hypo, you may not be able to think clearly enough to treat yourself. You may experience one or more of the following symptoms:
- Difficulty concentrating.
- Feeling disorientated.
- Acting out of character.
- Being aggressive.
- Being uncooperative.
- Blurred vision.
- Headache.

   If you are too confused to treat yourself, you need the help of people around you. This can be problematic, as you may be uncooperative and reluctant to accept help. However, relatives, friends, and workmates can become skilled at both recognizing the signs of a hypo and encouraging you to accept treatment.

   If you don't treat or receive treatment for your hypo and your blood glucose level continues to fall,

Myth OR TRUTH?

MYTH
If you have a hypo during the night and you don't wake up, you can die.

TRUTH
Hypos in the night usually wake you up, but even if you continue to sleep, your body will eventually correct your blood glucose level by converting glycogen in your liver into glucose and releasing it into your bloodstream. Excess insulin also wears off naturally in time. Hypos can occasionally be life-threatening if you have been drinking large amounts of alcohol on an empty stomach, because alcohol impairs this corrective mechanism.

you may lose consciousness. Getting to this stage normally takes quite a while after early warning symptoms start – up to 2 hours – but it may happen within 10 to 15 minutes of having the later symptoms.

Reduced awareness of symptoms

If you have a spell of frequent hypos – for example, three or four over a two-week period – your body gets used to the low blood glucose level and is less efficient at giving you early warning symptoms. By the time you realize you are having a hypo, your blood glucose level may have fallen below 3 millimoles per litre, at which point you are likely to find it difficult to treat the hypo yourself.

If you have had diabetes for years and have often had hypos, your body may not give you any early warning symptoms at all. Your only symptoms of a hypo may be confusion and disorientation, by which point it could be too late to treat the hypo yourself. This means that, if you don't receive help, you may lose consciousness. If you experience frequent hypos and

reduced awareness of symptoms, your health professional may suggest that you temporarily relax your diabetes control and allow your blood glucose level to rise above the ideal range of 4–7 millimoles per litre – to 10 or more millimoles per litre, for example. This provides a respite from hypos and can also help to restore your awareness of symptoms.

Treatment

There are two stages to treating a hypo: first, eating or drinking glucose as soon as possible, and, second, eating a more substantial carbohydrate-containing food to prevent your blood glucose level falling again. If you lose consciousness, you need help from someone else, which may include ambulance or hospital staff.

Initial treatment

As soon as you realize that you are having a hypo, you need to eat or drink something that is high in glucose – any of the following will start to raise your blood glucose level quickly (within 10–15 minutes):
- 3 glucose tablets – these are available from pharmacies.
- A high-energy sugar drink, ordinary cola, or lemonade.
- 2 teaspoons of sugar dissolved in water.
- 1 dose or 10g of glucose or dextrose gel (available from pharmacies).

If you take insulin or insulin-stimulating tablets, you should carry an emergency supply of glucose with

> **If you have had diabetes for years and have often had hypos, your body may not give you any early warning symptoms at all.**

My experience

"Over the years I've learned not to eat too much food when I have a hypo – I find 15–20 grams of carbohydrate is enough. This prevents my blood glucose getting too high afterwards." LOUISE

COMMENT It takes experience to know how much carbohydrate you need for the secondary treatment of a hypo. If you eat too much, you may get hyperglycaemia. Checking your blood glucose level when you feel better will tell you if what you have taken has been enough to correct your hypo.

Q **If I pass out during a hypo in a public place and I'm not with my family or friends, how will anyone know what's wrong with me?**

A Ambulance crew or hospital staff would automatically test your blood glucose level to work out whether hypoglycaemia is the cause of your unconsciousness. If you take insulin or insulin-stimulating tablets, always carrying identification giving details of your diabetes and treatment, such as an identification card or a piece of jewellery, will ensure that you are treated accurately and as quickly as possible.

you at all times. Apart from the list above, you may find a particular form and amount of glucose that suits you better, but remember that some glucose-rich food and drinks, such as chocolate or milky drinks with sugar, also contain fat, which slows down their absorption into your bloodstream.

Secondary treatment

After taking glucose, you need to eat something more substantial that contains carbohydrate. This could be:
● A sandwich.
● A piece of toast.
● A piece of fruit.
● 2–3 biscuits.
● A bowl of cereal.
  The exact amount of food you need depends on the circumstances of your hypo. For example, you may need several slices of toast if you won't be eating again for some time, or one biscuit if you are having a meal shortly. This

carbohydrate-containing food prevents your blood glucose level falling again after your body has used up the glucose you took previously. If you have a hypo just before a meal, take the initial treatment and let the meal act as the secondary treatment.

If you lose consciousness

If you are unconscious or losing consciousness, it is dangerous to try to eat or drink anything because you won't be able to swallow properly and you risk choking. Instead, you need an injection of either glucagon or glucose. Glucagon raises your blood glucose level by causing glycogen in your liver to be quickly converted into glucose and released into your bloodstream. An injection of glucagon will usually have an effect within 10 minutes. If you are

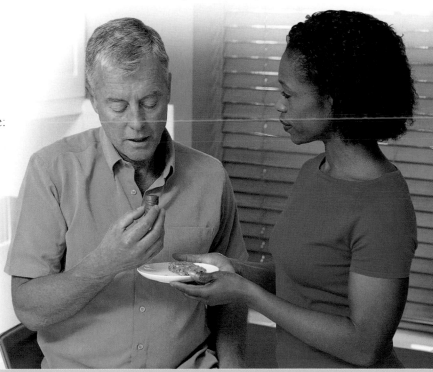

SECONDARY TREATMENT
Family or friends who know how to deal with hypoglycaemia will be able to help you when you need it, such as by giving you biscuits or a cereal bar as secondary treatment after you have taken glucose tablets.

at risk of losing consciousness during a hypo, your health professional can prescribe glucagon. A friend or relative can be shown how to give you the injection (see box, right). A glucose injection under your skin or into a vein in your arm can be given by ambulance crew or hospital staff. This also will help you regain consciousness within 5–10 minutes. Whether you receive a glucagon or glucose injection, you still need the secondary treatment of a carbohydrate snack or meal, as the glucose in your bloodstream will be used up quickly.

Getting help

If you take insulin or insulin-stimulating tablets, it's important to inform your family and friends about early warning symptoms, later symptoms, and the treatment of hypoglycaemia. This way, if you need help during a hypo, people know how to recognize this and what action to take. Other people who you may want to inform about the possibility of hypoglycaemia are work colleagues and people with whom you are drinking alcohol (alcohol increases the risk of a hypo, see pp.103–104). You may want a friend or relative to know how to test your blood glucose and, if you are prescribed glucagon, how to inject this (see box, right).

The recovery period

Even if you don't receive treatment for a hypo, your body eventually takes corrective action to raise the level of glucose in your blood. The glycogen in your liver is converted into glucose and released into your bloodstream to raise your blood glucose level. The effect of your insulin or insulin-stimulating tablets also wears off and this causes your blood glucose level to rise. So, although it is not ideal, even if you lose consciousness and there is no one to help you, you will regain consciousness naturally within an hour or two. There are exceptions to this, however: if you have a very large amount of insulin and/or alcohol in your bloodstream, this will cause your hypo to last much longer and be more severe.

In the recovery period following a hypo, your blood glucose level may become too high as a result of the

---

TREATING A HYPO – A CONSCIOUS PERSON

A family member, friend, or colleague who takes insulin or insulin-stimulating tablets may have a hypo from time to time. If the person is confused and unable to treat himself, you may need to treat him.

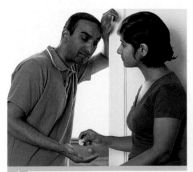

1 If a person is showing early symptoms of a hypo (see p.105), get him to test his blood glucose before treating his hypo. If he is showing later symptoms of a hypo (see p.105), give him 3 glucose tablets or a sugary drink.

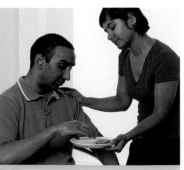

2 If he starts to feel better quickly, give him a carbohydrate snack, such as a biscuit. Don't give any food or drink to someone you suspect is losing consciousness – follow the procedure for dealing with someone who is unconscious (see box, right).

TREATING A HYPO – AN UNCONSCIOUS PERSON

If a hypo is untreated, and a person's blood glucose level continues to fall, he may lose consciousness. In this situation, you need to give a glucagon injection. Glucagon kits can be prescribed and should be stored in a fridge until needed.

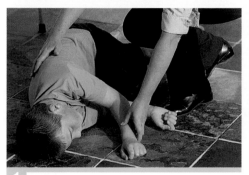

1 Put the person on his side, placing his arm and leg at right angles to his body. Tilt his head back to keep his airway clear.

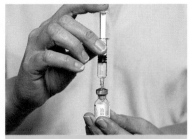

2 If you have access to a glucagon injection kit, remove the seal on the glucagon bottle. Uncap the needle, put it into the bottle, and inject the water from the syringe into the bottle.

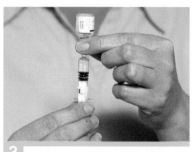

3 Rotate the bottle until all the glucagon powder has dissolved. Turn the bottle upside down and check the needle tip is in the solution. Pull the plunger to withdraw all the solution (it should fill the syringe to the 1ml mark).

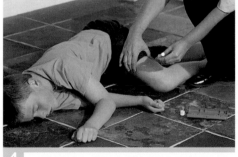

4 Insert the needle at a right angle into the person's thigh, buttock, or arm, and depress the plunger to inject. Withdraw the needle, press a tissue/swab against the injection site, and keep him in the recovery position until he is conscious.

In the recovery period following a hypo your blood glucose level may become too high as a result of the extra glucose that you have produced and consumed.

extra glucose that you have produced and consumed. This is known as "rebound hyperglycaemia" and it can happen shortly after a hypo or during the following 24 hours.

If you take rapid-acting insulin, you can use a small dose to correct rebound hyperglycaemia, but increasing your dose of other types of insulin may encourage further hypos because other insulins have a longer action. Instead, work out the cause of the hypo and take steps to prevent it happening again (see pp.102–105).

Even after you have treated a hypo and your blood glucose level is above 4 millimoles per litre, it may take you several hours to recover. In particular, you may feel unwell and find it difficult to concentrate.

Hyperglycaemia

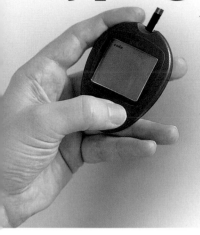

When you have diabetes, your body cells cannot take in glucose from your bloodstream, so the level of glucose in your blood remains high – this is known as hyperglycaemia. Your diabetes treatment is aimed at reducing hyperglycaemia and preventing your blood glucose becoming too high – above 7 millimoles per litre – on a regular basis. This helps protect you against short- and long-term complications. You can take action to treat hyperglycaemia according to its cause.

What is hyperglycaemia?

Hyperglycaemia is the term used to describe a raised blood glucose level (above 7 millimoles per litre). It is the main effect of untreated diabetes and so it may have been the symptoms of hyperglycaemia that led you to seek help when you were first diagnosed with diabetes.

Hyperglycaemia can not only make you feel unwell in the short-term, but also, if it happens frequently, it increases your risk of the long-term complications of diabetes. This is why a blood glucose level of 4–7 millimoles per litre is generally recommended for good diabetes control.

Although the main aim of diabetes treatment is to prevent hyperglycaemia, an occasional raised blood glucose level (7–10 millimoles per litre) is to be expected when you have diabetes. Even when you control your blood glucose level for most of the time, there are occasions when stress, illness, or not getting the right dose of insulin or tablets, for example, can raise your blood glucose level.

Hyperglycaemia can affect anyone with diabetes whether you take insulin, tablets, or manage your diabetes with healthy eating and physical activity.

The most obvious causes of hyperglycaemia are either an increase in the amount of food you eat or a decrease in the amount of activity you do.

Q **Can losing weight help me to prevent hyperglycaemia?**

A If you have a lot of body fat, your body needs a greater amount of insulin to control your blood glucose, so hyperglycaemia is more likely. If your BMI is in the recommended range (see p.46), your body is able to use insulin more efficiently than if you are overweight.

Causes and prevention

A key aspect of diabetes control is understanding what makes your blood glucose level rise and taking

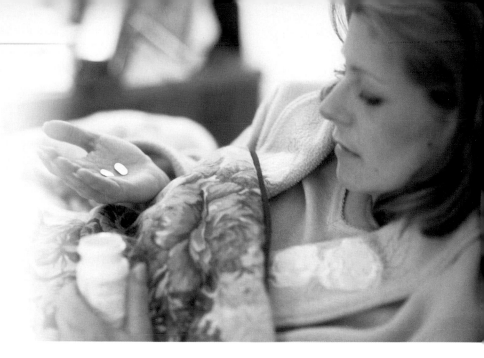

MONITORING DURING ILLNESS
When you are ill, your blood glucose level rises and can quickly get out of control. This is why it's very important to test your blood glucose level frequently and adjust your diabetes treatment accordingly.

action to prevent this happening. Regularly checking your blood glucose level to see if it is in the target range of 4–7 millimoles per litre can give you the information you need to prevent hyperglycaemia.

If you have a raised blood glucose level on a number of occasions – for example, if your test results are regularly 8–9 millimoles per litre – it's time to act quickly. Don't wait until you experience symptoms, because by this time your blood glucose level is likely to be 10 millimoles per litre or above.

■ **FOOD INTAKE/PHYSICAL ACTIVITY**
The most obvious causes of hyperglycaemia are either an increase in the amount of food you eat (resulting in extra glucose entering your bloodstream) or a decrease in the amount of activity you do (resulting in decreased use of glucose by your body cells). Eating certain types of food – those that

are high in sugar, for example – can also cause a raised blood glucose level. Ways of preventing hyperglycaemia include following healthy eating guidelines (see pp.30–43) and staying physically active (see pp.52–59).

■ **ILLNESS** When you are ill, glycogen in your liver is converted to glucose and released into your bloodstream. Increased amounts of the stress hormones cortisol and adrenaline are also produced and these stop your insulin working efficiently.

Both these processes cause your blood glucose level to rise. Frequent blood glucose monitoring is very important when you are ill because it enables you to react quickly and make the appropriate adjustments to your diabetes treatment.

■ **STRESS/HORMONAL CHANGES** Stress hormones can oppose the action of insulin in your body so that your blood glucose level rises as a

---

Practical tips

PREVENTING HYPERGLYCAEMIA

● Try to avoid overeating or, if you know you are going to eat more than usual, adjust your insulin or tablets (or be more active).

● Be aware of the effect of stress and other hormonal changes on your blood glucose level so that you can predict when you need to adjust your treatment.

● Don't stop taking your insulin/tablets when you are ill (especially if you have a vomiting illness) and monitor your blood glucose level frequently.

● Take your insulin or tablets every day and adjust the dose when necessary.

result. Also, when you are stressed you may overeat or eat less healthy types of food and this can cause your blood glucose to rise. If you are a woman, you may find that your blood glucose level rises at certain stages of your menstrual cycle (particularly just before periods). Hormonal changes during the menopause can also result in hyperglycaemia.

Some hormonal conditions (see p.17), such as Cushing's disease and acromegaly, are associated with hyperglycaemia, too, because they affect the efficiency of insulin. If you find that hormonal changes raise your blood glucose level, increase your frequency of blood glucose monitoring at the appropriate time – before your period, for example – and take action quickly.

■ **INSULIN/DIABETES TABLETS** If you haven't been able to take your insulin or tablets for any reason, your blood glucose level rises. Sometimes, you may have hyperglycaemia even though you have taken your insulin or tablets correctly – this suggests that you may need a different dose or type of insulin or tablet. If you have Type 2 diabetes that you manage with healthy eating and physical activity and your blood

> **If you are a woman, you may find that your blood glucose level rises at certain stages of your menstrual cycle.**

glucose level is frequently raised, you may need to start taking tablets – talk to your health professional.

Symptoms

The symptoms of hyperglycaemia are the same as those you may have had when your diabetes was first diagnosed (see pp.18–19). Possible symptoms include:

- Passing large amounts of urine frequently.
- Dry mouth, excessive thirst.
- Lack of energy.
- Weight loss.
- Blurred vision.
- Thrush and cystitis.

Hyperglycaemia may also be symptomless, especially if you have Type 2 diabetes or your body is used to a raised blood glucose level.

Treatment

You need to tailor your treatment of hyperglycaemia to its cause. This could mean decreasing your food intake, increasing your level of physical activity and/or increasing your insulin or tablet dosage (for information about adjusting your insulin dose, see pp.90–95). If you have Type 2 diabetes that you manage through healthy eating and physical activity, you may need to start taking tablets if your blood glucose level is consistently above 7 millimoles per litre. If you are ill, prompt treatment for your illness will limit the effect of hyperglycaemia (see pp.130–133).

My experience

"I know my blood glucose rises when I'm ill, even if I eat less, so I check my blood glucose 7–8 times a day and adjust my insulin accordingly." SOPHIE

COMMENT If you experience hyperglycaemia when you are unwell, it is important to adjust your treatment promptly when your blood glucose level is high, to prevent it becoming an emergency situation.

Whatever action you take to treat hyperglycaemia, test your blood glucose level frequently to check that it is returning to normal. If your blood glucose level falls as a result of increasing your dose of insulin or insulin-stimulating tablets, you may need to reduce the dosage once your blood glucose level is back in the recommended range.

If you cannot establish the cause of your hyperglycaemia or you are unsure how to go about treating it, talk to your health professional. Always treat hyperglycaemia promptly to avoid both short- and long-term complications.

Risks

An occasional, brief spell of hyperglycaemia may be uncomfortable, but is not likely to be harmful. However, a consistently high or rising blood glucose level can cause short- and long-term complications.

Short-term risks

If hyperglycaemia is untreated and your blood glucose level keeps rising (above 20 millimoles per litre) you may develop diabetic ketoacidosis if you have Type 1 diabetes or non-ketotic hyperosmolar state if you have Type 2 diabetes.

■ **DIABETIC KETOACIDOSIS (DKA)** If there is no insulin in your body, your body cells are unable to take in glucose from your bloodstream. This means that your body is deprived of its primary source of energy and is forced to break down fat as an alternative energy source. During fat breakdown, toxic by-products known as ketones are produced. An excessive amount of ketones in the body can make your blood highly acidic and cause symptoms such as nausea, vomiting, abdominal pain, and fruity-smelling breath (as a result of your body trying to expel ketones via your lungs). Untreated DKA can lead to coma and may occasionally be fatal. DKA is a medical emergency and needs to be treated in hospital. Treatment consists of an insulin infusion via a vein (see pp.134–135), intravenous fluids, potassium, and substances to correct the acidity of your blood.

■ **NON-KETOTIC HYPEROSMOLAR STATE** If you have Type 2 diabetes, you do not develop DKA because you still produce insulin, which means that your body has access to some glucose as an energy source and is not entirely dependent on fat as an alternative. However, severe hyperglycaemia can lead to excessive dehydration and occasionally a coma, which is known as a non-ketotic hyperosmolar state. This is also a very serious condition and needs to be treated in hospital.

Long-term risks

If your blood glucose level is raised over months and years, you have a greater risk of developing the long-term complications of diabetes such as eye, kidney, and heart disease, and damage to the nervous system (see pp.186–215).

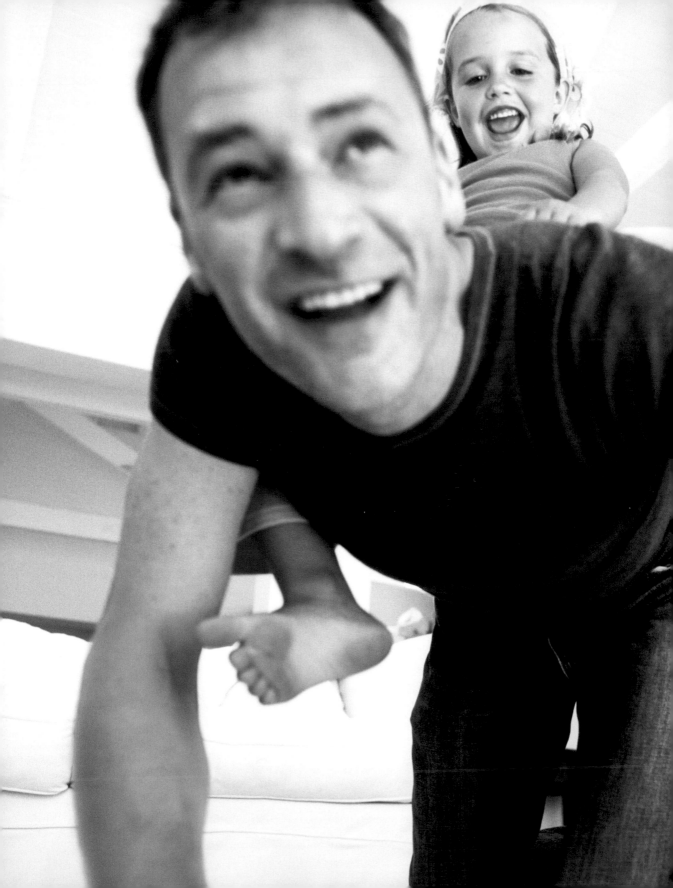

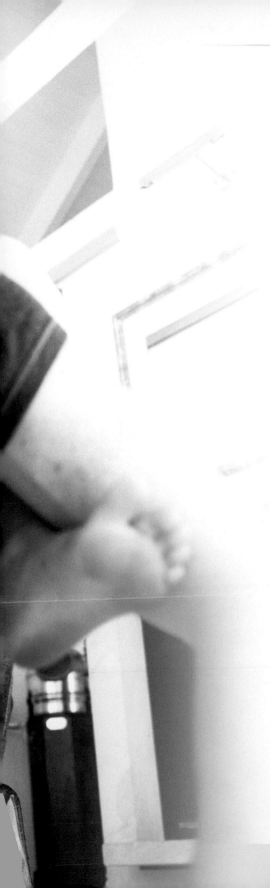

Living with diabetes

In most cases, diabetes is a lifelong condition, so it's essential to learn how to incorporate diabetes care into your daily life. Diabetes affects many aspects of your day-to-day life – from working to driving; from going on holiday to having sex. In all these instances, being informed and planning ahead will help you to anticipate and prevent problems.

Looking after yourself when you have diabetes includes taking care of your feet daily, and making sure that you take extra care of your diabetes when you are ill. Going into hospital may also mean you need a change in your diabetes management.

If you are a woman with diabetes, there are times when you need to be extra careful about monitoring your blood glucose level and tailoring your treatment to the results. Conception and pregnancy are times when tight control of your diabetes is essential. Gestational diabetes (diabetes that occurs during pregnancy) also needs careful treatment.

Living with diabetes involves regular contact with health professionals who provide help and support. It's useful to plan ahead before your appointments, so that you can get the most from your health care.

Day-to-day life

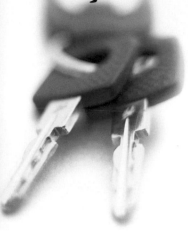

Looking after your diabetes every single day can require an effort of will, and learning how to motivate yourself to keep going is very important. Diabetes might affect you in your line of work, when driving a vehicle, and when travelling, and knowing how to deal with different situations will make it far less likely that diabetes will restrict you. Diabetes also affects the people you are close to, your relationships, and specific aspects of women's health and pregnancy.

Staying motivated

Diabetes is very different from a short-term illness, for which you might need, for example, a course of antibiotics, a short stay in hospital, or even an operation. In such circumstances, you expect the treatment to cure your illness and return you to full health, which helps motivate you to do whatever is necessary to recover. Once you have diabetes, unless it is gestational diabetes, you have it for life. Any care or treatment you receive is designed not to cure you but to prevent short-term problems, such as uncomfortable symptoms of hyperglycaemia, and the long-term complications of diabetes that could develop over years to come. While you can do much to protect yourself against complications, there is no guarantee that you won't develop problems at some point in your life. All this means that caring for your diabetes day after day requires lots of motivation. Feelings of despondency about the amount of effort you have to put in are entirely normal. Developing coping strategies to see you through the difficult times can help you to keep going.

Coping in the long term

There are a number of obstacles, perceived or real, that might get in the way of your diabetes care, such as:
- Being unable to identify when your blood glucose level is creeping up, because you still feel well.
- Not finding time to monitor your blood glucose level.

My experience

"Sometimes I feel like I'm in a straitjacket – I get sick and tired of caring for my diabetes and there are never any holidays." JOE

COMMENT You may feel that looking after your diabetes is a burden. If you feel trapped, taking time to identify your specific worries and devising a plan of action to overcome obstacles can help to refresh your motivation.

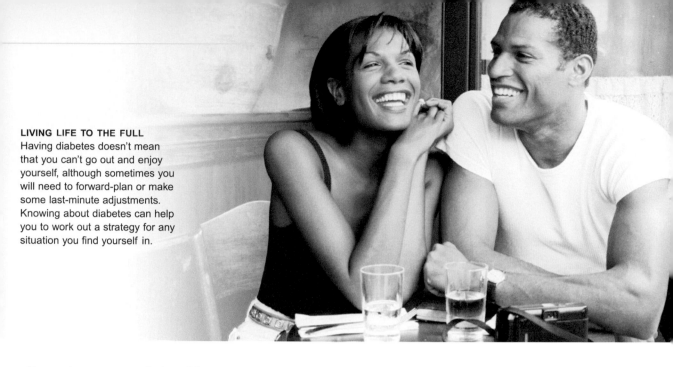

LIVING LIFE TO THE FULL
Having diabetes doesn't mean that you can't go out and enjoy yourself, although sometimes you will need to forward-plan or make some last-minute adjustments. Knowing about diabetes can help you to work out a strategy for any situation you find yourself in.

- Forgetting to, or not being able to, take your medication when you are supposed to.
- Having to eat what everyone else eats, healthy or not.
- Fitting in with others; not wanting to upset them.
- Not wanting to be different.
- Becoming fed up with your day-to-day routine.
- Feeling as though nothing you do makes a difference to your blood glucose level.

One way of tackling such obstacles is to follow a four-step action plan to help you make positive changes. Start by identifying the obstacle, explore how it makes you feel, consider ways to solve it, and finally decide what you will do to overcome it.

■ **WHAT GETS IN THE WAY?** Write down all the times when you find it difficult to look after your diabetes, and try to identify what exactly is getting in the way.

■ **HOW DOES IT MAKE YOU FEEL?** Consider how you feel about situations that prevent you from looking after your diabetes. For example, if your feelings are negative, acknowledging this can be a very important step.

■ **WHAT ARE YOUR OPTIONS?** Think about what you could do to change things for the better. You might have some ideas about this already. Visualize what you would like to happen and what options you have to bring this about.

■ **WHAT ARE YOU GOING TO DO?** Plan how you are going to bring about change. The more specific your plan, the more likely you are to achieve it. For example, if you want to lose weight, setting yourself a target and a time scale and then breaking them down into chunks will help you identify a weekly weight loss target. Then work out what changes to make on a daily basis to achieve this.

Write down all the times when you find it difficult to look after your diabetes, and try to identify what exactly is getting in the way.

If you want to remember to take your tablets more regularly, for example, the first step is to set a realistic target of how many days a week you will take all your tablets. The next step is to work out how you are going to achieve this on each of these days. To help you plan, ask yourself the following questions:

- What exactly are you going to do?
- When exactly will you start?
- Do you need to do anything to prepare for it beforehand?
- What will get in the way of you achieving it?
- How can you reduce the chances of anything getting in the way?

Ask yourself if what you have planned is really possible. If not, set yourself smaller targets to ensure success. Monitor your progress to check that you are on target for success. If you are succeeding, you need to congratulate yourself. If you haven't quite succeeded, try not to get disheartened. Instead, review your options, identify one that is realistic and achievable, and set yourself a different goal and timescale. If you are still struggling to achieve your goals, you could ask for the help of someone close to you, perhaps to monitor your progress or to talk through whatever it is that you find difficult. Changing behaviour takes time, so be prepared – and keep trying.

> **If you manage your diabetes with healthy eating and physical activity, there should be no restrictions on the type of work that you do.**

Work

There are very few jobs that you cannot do if you have diabetes. If you manage your diabetes with healthy eating and physical activity, there should be no restrictions on the type of work that you do. If you manage your diabetes with tablets or insulin injections, there is only a small number of jobs that you are not eligible to apply for (see below). By keeping your diabetes well controlled, you can make sure that it does not affect your performance at work. It may even have a positive influence on colleagues as they see you managing your job and your diabetes without any problems.

Applying for jobs

If you take insulin for your diabetes, you will not be able to join the police, the armed forces, or the fire brigade, nor can you fly commercial aircraft. In addition, you won't be eligible to apply for jobs that involve working offshore, including on ferries and passenger liners, become a diver or a jockey, or drive trains. If you take insulin, you won't usually be able to drive large goods vehicles (LGV), or passenger carrying vehicles

My experience

"My husband really understands my concerns and the issues that frighten me. He sits down and talks to me about how we can deal with things together." SOPHIE

COMMENT Having the support of someone close to you can help you cope more easily when times are difficult. You could ask your partner to monitor your progress if you are trying to make changes, or simply to talk through any aspects of your diabetes care that are worrying you.

> **Q** Is there anything that I can do if I believe that I am being turned down for a job simply because I have diabetes?
>
> **A** If you think that you are being denied a job because you have diabetes, your potential employer should be able to provide concrete reasons why the position would not be suitable for you. If you believe that their reasons are discriminatory, you can contact Diabetes UK to discuss your situation. The organization may provide support if you decide to pursue your case. There have been several successful court cases in which people with diabetes have proved that they can do their jobs just as well as people without diabetes.

(PCV), although there are exceptions (see p.121).

Most of these restrictions apply if you take tablets for your diabetes, though you may be able to drive trains, LGVs, and PCVs.

When applying for a job, you are not legally obliged to inform your potential employers that you have diabetes unless you are asked about your health, in which case stating that you have diabetes and giving details of your treatment is sufficient.

If you are not asked about your health, you may feel reluctant to volunteer the information, especially if you think you are less likely to be offered the job as a result. However, telling your employer may enable you to eat when you need to at work without it causing any difficulty and have time off if you need it for medical reasons. You should also tell an employer that you have diabetes if you take insulin or insulin-stimulating tablets and you are responsible for other people's safety.

Some potential employers may have justifiable concerns about your safety when carrying out certain tasks, such as driving, operating heavy machinery, or working at heights. In these circumstances you could be in danger if your medication puts you at risk of a hypo and you were to have a hypo with very little warning.

However, if you can demonstrate that your blood glucose is well controlled, through self-monitoring results and medical reports if necessary, these jobs should still be accessible to you.

You have the option of registering as disabled when you have diabetes. Some companies try to employ a percentage of people who are registered disabled, so, in some cases, your diabetes might help you to win the job you want.

On the other hand, you may not view your diabetes as a disability, or you may feel that it would not be to your advantage to register. If you are unsure whether or not to register as disabled, ask your health professional or contact Diabetes UK for advice.

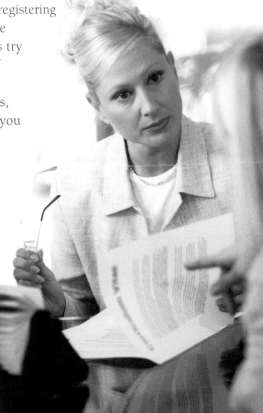

ATTENDING INTERVIEWS
Potential employers are unlikely to discriminate against you when you have diabetes, especially if you talk to them openly about how diabetes affects you and what can be expected of you.

Continuing in your existing job

If you discover that you have diabetes while already working in a restricted field of employment, you will not necessarily be dismissed (although starting to take insulin will disqualify you from holding a commercial pilot's licence or LGV or PCV licence).

Whether an employer will allow you to continue in your position will depend on the type of work you do, the extent to which diabetes affects it, and on the risk to yourself and others.

Blood glucose control

However busy your job, caring for your diabetes is important if you are to perform well; a high blood glucose level could affect your ability to perform by making you feel unwell and a low level could lead to hypoglycaemia.

Whether you have a regular schedule or one that changes from one day to the next, your diabetes should not hold you back, provided that you can devise a routine to suit your diabetes and fit into your working day.

If the job that you do is quite unpredictable or involves a lot of physical activity, you may need to check your blood glucose level three to four times during the working day. You may also need to find time for snacks or extra food at mealtimes. If you need to take insulin or tablets at mealtimes, it's a good idea to keep a supply at work, along with some emergency hypo remedies, such as glucose tablets or glucose drinks, if you take insulin or insulin-stimulating tablets.

If you know that you have hypos without warning, it's important that your colleagues know what they can do to help (see pp.106–109). Tell them what supplies you have for treating a hypo, where you keep them, and what colleagues might need to do if you are unable to deal with the hypo yourself.

If colleagues are concerned about your hypos and their effect on your ability to do your job, your health professional should be able to work with you and your employer to find a way of dealing with your diabetes that enables you to get on with your job effectively and stay well. You could discuss a change of insulin or tablet dose or type to suit your work pattern better, or identify ways of recognizing hypos early.

Driving

You can obtain a licence for most types of vehicle when you have diabetes, which means that, along with other motorists, you are responsible for your own safety and that of other road users. For this reason, it is very important to take precautions to avoid hypoglycaemia while driving. If you do become hypo at the wheel, you should know exactly what action to take so as not to endanger yourself or other people. You should also ensure that your vision is good enough to drive safely (see p.195).

Practical tips

COPING WITH SHIFT WORK

- Monitor your blood glucose to find out what effect working shifts has on your diabetes, so that you can adjust your tablets or insulin accordingly.

- Remember that insulin and tablets need to be taken in relation to your food intake as opposed to the time of day.

- If break times or the type of work you do are subject to change at short notice, make sure you always have glucose and carbohydrate snacks with you if you take insulin or insulin-stimulating tablets.

- Ask your health professional for advice if you think you need a different tablet or insulin to suit your shift pattern.

You will need to notify your car insurance company if you have diabetes. However, an insurance company cannot refuse you insurance or increase your premium unless it has evidence that you are a higher-risk driver; well-controlled diabetes does not put you at added risk, so your premiums should not go up automatically. If you encounter any problems, you can obtain driving insurance quotes through Diabetes UK (see p.218).

If you take tablets or insulin for your diabetes, you will also need to inform the Driving and Vehicle Licensing Agency (DVLA) that you have diabetes. If your diabetes is treated with healthy eating and physical activity only, you do not need to contact the DVLA.

What the DVLA needs to know

If you take tablets to manage your diabetes, the DVLA will not restrict your licence in any way. If you take insulin, your licence will be granted on the basis of how well controlled your diabetes is. The DVLA will require you to fill in a form about your diabetes and provide contact details for your GP or health professional. You will need to renew your licence at least every three years if you take insulin, and more frequently if the DVLA has any concerns about your ability to drive. If you take insulin, you are not allowed to drive LGVs or PCVs, although some long-standing licence

My experience

"I don't want to feel different, but some people are ignorant about diabetes and think I have some major disability that will prevent me from doing my job properly." SHELLEY

COMMENT Your colleagues may know little about diabetes, or they may know someone with diabetes and expect you to be the same. Taking time to explain how diabetes affects you as an individual will dispel misconceptions and lessen some of your own frustrations.

holders may be exempt. If you drive a vehicle between 3.5–7.5 tonnes, your application to continue is considered. Your health professional or the DVLA will give you more information.

To maintain the validity of your current licence, you should inform the DVLA in writing as soon as possible after starting any treatment for your diabetes. If you are applying for a licence for the first time and you have tablet- or insulin-treated diabetes, you should notify the DVLA at this point.

If you have gestational diabetes and you start taking insulin (see pp.144–145), you should inform the DVLA. You can keep your current licence unless you have, or are reported to have, hypos without warning. If you are still taking insulin six weeks after having your baby, you will need to notify the DVLA again.

Safety at the wheel

Driving while you are hypoglycaemic is categorized as driving under the influence of drugs (insulin), dangerous driving, or driving without due care and attention. This means that you

An insurance company cannot refuse you insurance or increase your premium unless it has evidence that you are a higher-risk driver; well-controlled diabetes does not put you at added risk …

Myth OR TRUTH?

MYTH
When you're on holiday, you can also take a break from your diabetes.

TRUTH
You may be more relaxed about food and drink on holiday, but you can't afford to forget about your diabetes – unusual routines and heat can cause your blood glucose level to change more than usual. You will need to keep an eye on your blood glucose level and perhaps adjust your insulin or tablet doses to prevent it from getting too high or low. You should also take swift action if you get a holiday stomach upset as well as take particular care to look after your feet.

My experience

"When I'm packing to go away, it really annoys me that I have to leave space in my suitcase for all my diabetes equipment. I know I need it, but I still resent it!" JOE

COMMENT When you have diabetes you may have extra luggage, but it is worth being well prepared because you may not be able to obtain the equipment you need while you are away.

could lose your licence if you are stopped by the police or have an accident while you are hypoglycaemic.

You are at risk of hypos only if you take insulin-stimulating tablets or insulin injections, so in both cases you will need to take the following precautions when you drive.

- Always test your blood glucose before you drive, to check that it is at a safe level.
- Test your blood glucose level at least every 2 hours during a long journey.
- Keep supplies of food and drink to treat a hypo (see p.106) close by (not in the boot of the car).
- Carry identification.

If you have a hypo while you are driving, pull over immediately, stop the car, and treat the hypo. Make it clear that you do not intend to carry on driving until you have recovered by taking your keys out of the ignition and moving to the passenger seat until you are better. You should not drive again until your blood glucose level is above 4 millimoles per litre and you feel well.

If you know you do not experience clear warning signs during a hypo, you will need to be much stricter

about driving by stopping to test your blood glucose frequently or by travelling with people who will quickly recognize if you are starting to have a hypo.

Holidays and travel

When you are away from home, be it on holiday or for business reasons, a different environment or routine is likely to have an effect on your diabetes management. There are a number of practicalities to consider before you go. Long distance travel, changes in temperature, and different foods, drinks, or activities can all affect your blood glucose. The better you can plan ahead and anticipate any potential problems, the more enjoyable and successful your trip will be.

Before you go

Check that you will be insured for any diabetes-related problems while you are away. Make sure that your travel insurance does not exclude pre-existing conditions such as diabetes and that you are covered for any hospital stay and your return journey.

Wherever you're going, you will need to take more than enough diabetes equipment and medication for the trip. Even if you are travelling within the UK, it can be difficult to get hold of replacement equipment or medication at short notice. Abroad, many tablets, insulin, and blood-testing strips are named differently and may even be packaged in different sizes or strengths. Having plenty of your own supplies means that you can always stay in control of your treatment.

If you will be flying to your destination, ask your health professional to write a letter explaining to the authorities that your diabetes equipment needs to remain in your hand luggage. It is very important to keep some equipment with you in case your baggage is lost. Also, insulin can freeze in the hold of an aircraft, making it ineffective. A letter from your health professional will prevent your fingerpricking lancets or insulin needles being confiscated at the airport. It's a good idea to put some supplies in a travelling companion's hand luggage, too, in case yours becomes separated from you.

Before you travel, find out what types of food will be available at your destination so that you can take any extra foods you may need with you. Bear in mind that travelling across time zones can affect your blood glucose level, your eating pattern, and the timing of your treatment. Thinking in advance about when you expect to fly, arrive, and when your meal times are likely to be will help you plan what measures to take and what food to carry with you in case there is none available when you need it.

CHECKING IN FOR A FLIGHT
When you check in, let airline staff know that you have diabetes medication and equipment in your hand luggage. If necessary show them your letter from your health professional.

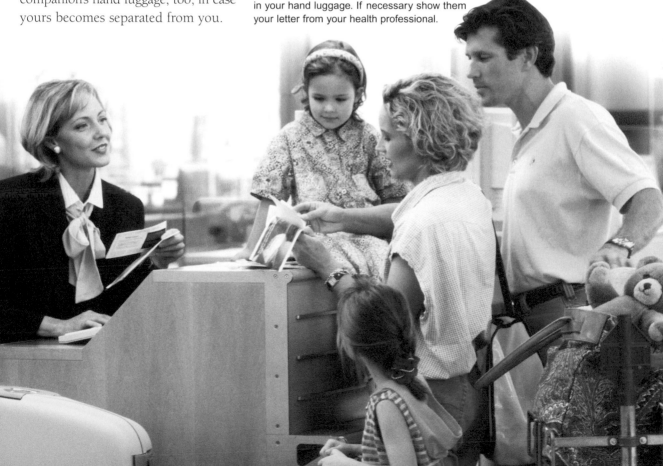

When you pack, include the following:
● Insulin or tablets – at least double the supply you need.
● Blood glucose monitoring meter, lancets, and strips.
● Cool bag or flask, if you take insulin.
● Hypo treatments, if you need them.
● Food supplies.
● Identification.
● Information about how to manage your diabetes when you are unwell.
● Your health professional's contact details.
● Insurance details.

Looking after your equipment and medication

All your equipment and medicines should be stored in a cool, dry place. Unopened insulin bottles, cartridges,

HEAT AND DEHYDRATION
Hot weather can cause dehydration, as can a high blood glucose level. A combination of the two will you make you feel very unwell. In a hot climate, you should drink plenty of water or other sugar-free fluids, and monitor your blood glucose level regularly.

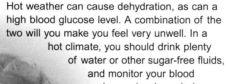

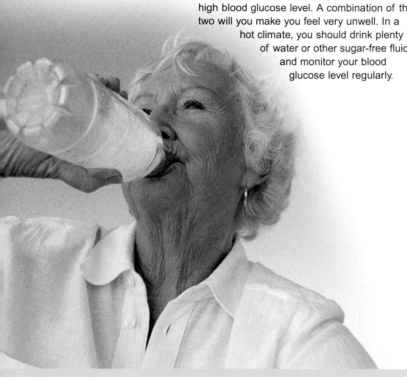

or disposable injection devices should be kept in a fridge (at a temperature of 2–8°C/36–47°F). If you don't have access to a fridge at your destination or if you are travelling long haul, you will need to use a cool bag or flask to store your insulin. If you are flying, make sure that you keep your insulin with you in your hand luggage – it can freeze in the hold of a plane.

The insulin you are currently using will be safe at a room temperature of up to 25°C (77°F) for up to a month, provided you keep it out of direct sunlight. In higher temperatures, you will need to keep it in a cool bag, flask, or water, or wrapped in cool cloths. In cool climates, you will need to keep your insulin above 2°C (36°F), either on your person or using a flask.

Crossing time zones

When you are travelling across time zones, blood glucose testing every few hours is essential to find out whether you need any extra medication or food. You may find that your blood glucose level is erratic for 24 hours.

Hypoglycaemia is always a concern when crossing time zones, but because you are probably using less energy than usual while travelling, the risk is somewhat reduced. If you are feeling excited or stressed, the hormones you produce will also have the effect of raising your blood glucose level. If, during the journey, your level is a little higher than you would like, you can rectify this when you arrive at your destination. Travelling across time zones is less problematic if you are taking rapid-acting insulin (see pp.84–85) or tablets (see pp.76–81). If you are not using this type of medication and you anticipate problems when travelling, ask your health professional whether a change in medication would benefit you.

While you are away

Hot weather increases your circulation, so can speed up the rate at which insulin or tablets are absorbed into your bloodstream. (This can also happen if you have a massage or use hot jacuzzis, spas, or sunbeds.) Therefore, if you take insulin or insulin-stimulating tablets, heat can make you prone to hypoglycaemia. You may need to reduce your dose or have extra carbohydrate snacks or eat more carbohydrate at mealtimes to make hypos less likely.

If you become very cold, for example while skiing, your circulation will slow down and so your insulin or tablets may take longer than usual to work. Wearing warm clothes and being physically active are likely to counteract this, so your blood glucose level shouldn't rise too high. Whatever the weather, it's important to keep testing your blood glucose to deal with any temperature-related problems.

While you are away, you may want to experiment with new foods, drinks, and activities. Again, testing will enable you to find out what effects these may have on your blood glucose and help you keep it in the recommended range. To avoid stomach upsets, which may cause your blood glucose level to rise, be careful about what you consume. Eat food that has been cooked properly and not left standing, drink bottled mineral or spring water, and eat only well-washed salad and peeled fruit.

If you take part in any strenuous physical activity, remember that it may affect your blood glucose many hours later, so you need to know how to prevent hypoglycaemia in these circumstances (see pp.56–59).

Don't forget to look after your feet. It's all too easy to scrape your foot in the sea, or to develop blisters when you're sightseeing or on hot sand, and not notice any injury. Never wear new shoes for the first time on holiday – take your most comfortable shoes with you. Also, never go barefoot, even on the beach. Keeping your feet protected by footwear at all times will reduce the risk of injury. Check your feet frequently and take action if necessary (see pp.128–130).

> If you become very cold, for example while skiing, your circulation will slow down and so your insulin or tablets may take longer than usual to work.

My experience

"I have travelled the world 3 times, lived in the desert, gone backpacking, ice climbing, and cycling. You can do whatever you want – just manage your diabetes as you go along." JOE

COMMENT Diabetes does not have to prevent you from going anywhere you want to go or doing any activity you want to do. Planning ahead and thinking carefully about how you will manage your diabetes in different circumstances will ensure your trip is successful.

"I always had the fear that no man would ever want to marry me because I had diabetes. But I told my husband-to-be when I met him, and it never put him off!" SOPHIE

COMMENT You may be wary of telling a new partner that you have diabetes, especially if you expect him or her to react badly. However, it's important to be honest from the start, even if you expect the worst – you could be surprised by the positive response you receive.

Sex and relationships

Diabetes has implications not only for you, but also for your partner and needs to be considered when you have sex, both in terms of the effect of sexual activity on your blood glucose level and the possibility of pregnancy. Reliable contraception is all-important when you are female and have diabetes, because you need very good blood glucose control before you conceive and during pregnancy.

TALKING TO EACH OTHER
Diabetes can give rise to conflicting emotions within a relationship, often due to love, concern, stress, or fear. Sharing your feelings with your partner, ideally at times when neither of you is feeling pressured, will help you to understand each other's point of view.

Diabetes can also affect sexual function, most commonly in men, but also in women.

Finding ways of involving your partner if he or she wants to feel included can help to alleviate concerns when they arise. For example, you might want to take your partner to your annual diabetes review so that he or she can gain a better understanding of any treatment you need. There may, however, be aspects of your diabetes care that you prefer to manage on your own. Be honest with your partner if this is how you feel – it is your diabetes, your health, and your decision as to how you deal with it.

Blood glucose control

Because sexual activity can use up a lot of energy, it should be treated in the same way as other types of physical activity (see pp.56–58). There are also a number of additional practicalities to consider. If you take insulin or insulin-stimulating tablets, there is a risk that sex, like any form of strenuous activity, could cause hypoglycaemia. Testing your blood glucose level before you have sex and again a few hours later will help you to gauge the effect and decide whether you need to take any measures to prevent a hypo. You may find that you need to either reduce your

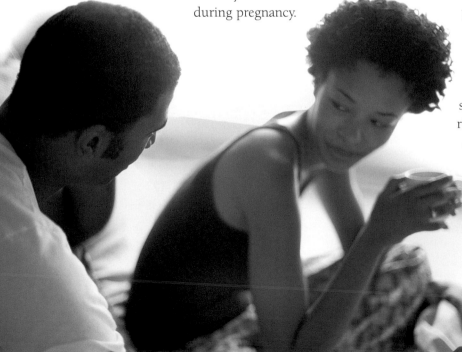

insulin dose beforehand or eat more in order to keep your blood glucose level in the ideal range.

Keep some high-carbohydrate snacks or drinks to hand, so that if you have a hypo you will be able to deal with it quickly (see p.106). It's important to remember that your blood glucose level can fall several hours after physical activity, so you should be prepared for this eventuality, too. Your partner may need to give you a glucagon injection if you become too hypo to take action yourself.

Contraception

When you have diabetes, it is extremely important that pregnancy is planned, because good blood glucose control is essential from the moment of conception (see pp.138–147 for more information on diabetes and pregnancy). You can use any method of contraception, so it's important to choose the one that will be most reliable for you.

Oral contraceptive pills contain low doses of hormones, which may have a small effect on your blood glucose level, but they are among the most reliable forms of contraception and are completely safe to take if you have diabetes. If your blood glucose level fluctuates a lot while taking an oral contraceptive, you can adjust your insulin or tablets to compensate.

Sexual function

Problems with sexual function or performance are not unique to people with diabetes. However, erectile

Q **Does having diabetes mean that sex can never be spontaneous?**

A You should test your blood glucose level before having sex, as with before any physical activity, but there are always occasions when you want to be spontaneous. In general, having spontaneous sex (without testing beforehand) at times when you know that your blood glucose level will be low, is unwise. If you haven't tested your blood glucose level before having sex, have a high-glucose snack directly after sex and test your blood glucose, too.

dysfunction (see pp.213–215) is recognized as a complication of diabetes in men. Sexual function has been less widely researched in women, but it is thought that diabetes can affect a woman's sexual response. Vaginal dryness is a fairly common complaint, while some women might find sex painful, lose interest in sex, or be unable to achieve an orgasm as they used to.

Problems with sexual performance may have physical or psychological roots. If you are experiencing difficulties, you could talk to your health professional about treatment options. If there is a physical cause, you may be offered treatments such as vaginal lubricants if you are a woman, or drugs that stimulate your erection if you are man who is experiencing difficulty with this. Some drugs may also be useful for women, although this form of treatment is still being researched. Counselling can help you to deal with psychological issues.

When you have diabetes, it is extremely important that pregnancy is planned, because good blood glucose control is essential from the moment of conception.

Looking after yourself

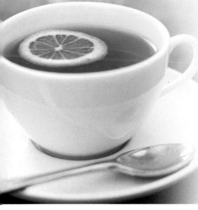

When you have diabetes, there are aspects of your health that need special attention. For example, your feet should be checked daily. Because common illnesses can affect diabetes control, it's important to take steps to keep your blood glucose level in the target range and help speed up your recovery. Being admitted to hospital may also disrupt your diabetes management, so knowing what to do in this situation is also important.

Footcare

Over time, diabetes can have an impact on the efficiency of your blood circulation and nervous system, which can affect many areas of the body. Your feet are particularly susceptible to problems caused by poor circulation and nerve damage because they are furthest from your heart, and the main nerves in your legs are very long. You are, therefore, more prone to foot ulcers and other injuries, which can become infected and lead to serious problems. Also, because nerve damage can cause numbness in such extremities, you may not experience the soreness that would normally alert you to any injuries.

In extreme cases, an injury may take a long time to heal or can even lead to your foot or leg being amputated. This is why your feet and circulation are examined at your annual review (see p.26).

In between reviews, you can take good care of your feet yourself by checking them every day. You can also help to prevent injuries by, most importantly, never walking barefoot – not even in your own home and particularly when you are in unfamiliar surroundings. Wear something on your feet indoors and always on a beach to avoid burning your feet on hot sand.

Your daily routine

You should wash and dry your feet thoroughly every day, and apply an unperfumed moisturizing cream afterwards. You should then check the top and sides of your feet carefully, looking for any tender, bruised or hard, cracked, or callused skin, and the beginnings of blisters or corns.

Check the soles of your feet, too. (If this is hard for you to do, ask someone to help you.) Cut your toenails when you need to. However, if you know that you have reduced

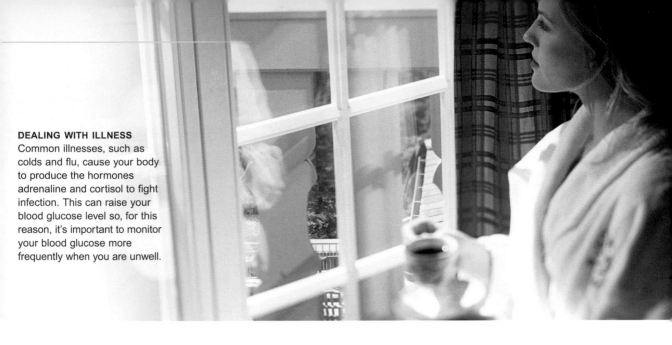

DEALING WITH ILLNESS
Common illnesses, such as colds and flu, cause your body to produce the hormones adrenaline and cortisol to fight infection. This can raise your blood glucose level so, for this reason, it's important to monitor your blood glucose more frequently when you are unwell.

feeling or circulation in your feet, check with your health professional that it is still alright for you to cut your own nails. If you can't bend to cut your nails, or they are too thick to cut, ask someone to help you.

Dealing with problems

Although you can treat some minor foot problems yourself, keep in mind that some fairly ordinary foot conditions, such as corns and hard skin, require the attention of a health professional.

■ **MINOR PROBLEMS** Athlete's foot can be treated at home with a fungal powder or cream. Keep the skin clean and dry, especially between your toes.

If you have a small blister, don't pop it and avoid putting pressure on it. If the blister pops, cover it with a piece of gauze and tape, and keep checking it to make sure it heals.

Verrucae will normally go away without treatment in time, but they may cause an imbalance of pressure on your feet, especially if your nerves have been affected. Being assessed by a health professional will give you the information you need and enable you to treat them appropriately.

■ **WHEN TO GET HELP** Most other foot problems require professional care, so you need to contact your health professional if you develop any of the following conditions:

● Corns – never treat these yourself, either by cutting them or rubbing

> **Q** Why all the fuss about my feet just because I have diabetes? Surely I would be able to tell if there was something wrong?

> **A** Sometimes foot problems start because the nerves supplying the feet have been damaged. If this applies to you, you may not feel a small injury, or notice a problem developing until it becomes serious. The only way to tell if anything is wrong is to check your feet all over every day. If you can't do this yourself, ask someone to do it for you.

You can help to prevent injuries by never walking barefoot – not even in your own home and particularly when you are in unfamiliar surroundings.

LOOKING AFTER YOUR FEET

A good foot-care regimen will help you to keep your feet healthy and enable you to notice potential problems early on. Carry out this procedure every day, allowing plenty of time to thoroughly check your feet for injuries and problems.

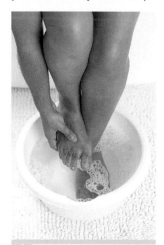

1 Wash your feet daily in warm water, using a mild soap. Avoid soaking your feet for more than 10 minutes, however, because this can dry out the skin.

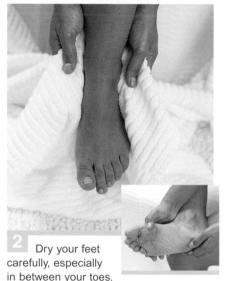

2 Dry your feet carefully, especially in between your toes. Now check for tender areas, bruising, and cuts or hard or cracked skin on the top and on the soles of your feet.

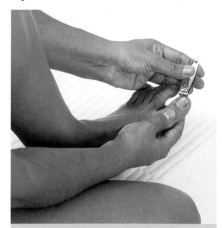

3 Trim your toenails when you need to. Cut them to the shape of and level with the end of your toe. Don't cut them too short and don't stick sharp instruments down the side of a nail.

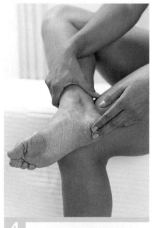

4 Apply an unperfumed moisturizing cream to your feet, paying attention to the skin between your toes and any hard skin on your soles.

them, and never use medicated corn plasters or dressings.
- Burns or injuries.
- A sore area that isn't healing.
- An ingrowing toenail.
- Bruising or discoloured areas on your feet with no apparent cause.
- Hard or cracked skin.
- New loss of feeling in any part of your foot – for example, if you can't feel a stone in your shoe.

It is important to get professional help if you can't look after your feet yourself and there is no one else to do it for you, or if you are concerned about your feet in any way, even if you think your worry is trivial.

Daily comfort

Don't wear tight or restrictive socks, stockings, or tights that rub or cramp your toes, and remember not to put your feet directly against a hot-water bottle, hot radiator, or heater, or near an open fire, as you may accidentally burn your feet if you can't feel the heat. Check your footwear daily to make sure there are no parts that are rubbing your feet, or sharp objects inside the shoe or sticking through the sole. Also, check the soles and uppers of your shoes for uneven wear that may be a clue to particular areas of pressure on your feet.

When you become ill

In itself, having diabetes does not make you more prone to common illnesses than anyone else. But if your diabetes is poorly controlled and your blood glucose level is consistently high, you may pick up infections more easily or simply feel unwell. This is because bacteria and viruses thrive when your blood glucose is consistently above 10 millimoles per litre. Any illness can affect your diabetes, particularly if it lasts for several days, or requires medical or hospital treatment. Blood glucose control can also affect the speed of your recovery.

The effect on your diabetes

Whatever type of diabetes you have, illness is likely to raise your blood glucose level. This is because part of your body's natural reaction to illness is to release more glucose into your bloodstream and to produce stress hormones such as adrenaline and cortisol. These hormones make your natural or injected insulin less efficient, which can cause hyperglycaemia, even if you are not eating anything.

One symptom of hyperglycaemia is dehydration, which can be aggravated by a high body temperature. Therefore, a sudden, acute illness, such as food poisoning with sickness and diarrhoea, and its combined effects of high blood glucose, dehydration, and infection can cause your diabetes to become seriously out of control and also affect other body processes.

If you have Type 1 diabetes, this situation may result in diabetic ketoacidosis (see p.113). If you have Type 2 diabetes, you might become severely dehydrated, which can

occasionally lead to coma (see p.113). Both these conditions require urgent hospital treatment.

Blood glucose control

You may not be ill very often, so it can be difficult to remember what effect illness has on your blood glucose level and how to respond. Next time you are unwell, write down what action you take to control your blood glucose and keep your notes to refer to again if you need to.

When you are ill, there are two golden rules to remember:
• Test your blood glucose level at least every four hours.
• Continue taking your insulin or tablets, even if you are not eating anything.

Your tests will tell you what effect your illness is having on your blood glucose level, while taking your tablets or insulin will help to combat the natural increase in blood glucose that illness causes. If you feel too ill to do blood glucose tests or even to think about your diabetes treatment, you need to ask a friend or family member to do it for you, or contact your health professional.

When you are ill, keeping your blood glucose level below 10 millimoles per litre will help your recovery. You may need to temporarily increase your dose of tablets or insulin to achieve this, and you can reduce the dose again when you feel better. If you have a longer illness, particularly when you are confined to bed for weeks or months,

Myth OR TRUTH?

MYTH
If you are not able to eat when you're ill, you should stop taking your tablets or insulin to prevent a hypo.

TRUTH
Your body produces glucose even if you are not eating when you are ill, and may produce more to give your body extra energy to recover from illness. You need to continue to take your tablets or insulin to keep your glucose level down. You may even need to increase your dose.

Whatever type of diabetes you have, illness is likely to raise your blood glucose level.

Drugs that you buy over the counter are safe to take when you have diabetes, although some may affect your blood glucose level.

keeping your blood glucose level in the normal range will help prevent complications arising.

If your body is particularly sensitive to insulin, illness can occasionally cause hypoglycaemia. If you have Type 1 diabetes and experience a "honeymoon period"– a period of up to two years after being diagnosed with diabetes when your pancreas makes some insulin again – your body will be sensitive to insulin during this time. Children may also experience a lower blood glucose level when unwell. In these circumstances, you may need to reduce your dose of tablets or insulin, but be careful that this doesn't make your blood glucose level rise too high.

Eating and drinking

Eating and drinking gives your body energy to combat your illness and limits the effects of an illness on your diabetes. You may also need small amounts of drinks containing glucose. If you can't eat, a day or two without food will not matter too much, but drinking plenty of sugar-free fluids throughout the day is essential. This helps to keep your temperature down and prevent dehydration if your blood glucose level is raised.

Diarrhoea and vomiting

Your body tries to get rid of anything it perceives as harmful, such as infected food, by expelling it from your system. Bouts of sickness and diarrhoea may be short-lived, but they can have a serious effect on your diabetes within a few hours.

■ **TYPE 1 DIABETES** If you become hyperglycaemic and dehydrated as a result of prolonged vomiting and diarrhoea, and you are not able to keep any food or fluids down, your body might develop ketones in large quantities. Ketones make you even more nauseous because they irritate your stomach, and they also affect the acid balance of your blood. If this happens, your organs are unable to function properly, which could lead to unconsciousness and even death. This condition is known as diabetic ketoacidosis (see p.113).

You can prevent diabetic ketoacidosis and serious illness by always taking your insulin, even if you are not eating, are being sick, or simply don't feel like injecting. You need to test your urine or blood for ketones using dipsticks or a blood glucose meter in order to assess the seriousness of your condition. If you have ketones, or if you have diarrhoea and vomiting that continues for more than 2–3 hours, contact your health professional. You may need to be treated in hospital.

■ **TYPE 2 DIABETES** You are not at risk of developing diabetic ketoacidosis if you have diarrhoea and vomiting, but your blood glucose level can still rise extremely high and you can become very dehydrated, which can lead to a coma (a condition known as hyperglycaemic non-ketotic hyperosmolar state, see p.113). If you are unable to take your tablets (if you have them) or to keep any fluids down, contact your health professional immediately, as you may need treatment for your dehydration, either at home or in hospital.

Over-the-counter medicines

Drugs that you buy over the counter are safe to use when you have diabetes, although some may affect your blood glucose level. Cough syrup, for example, may contain a lot of sugar, but as you only take a teaspoonful or two of syrup in a single dose, the effect on your blood glucose will be minimal. Ideally, ask your pharmacist to recommend a low-sugar product.

Long-term drug treatments

If you are prescribed drugs to treat a condition other than your diabetes, these might affect your blood glucose level. If a range of drugs is available to treat your condition, your doctor will choose the one that has least effect on your blood glucose. If there is only one drug treatment your doctor can prescribe and this is likely to affect your blood glucose, the type or dose of insulin or tablets you take for your diabetes may need to change.

High blood pressure

Certain tablets used to treat high blood pressure, including thiazide diuretics such as bendroflumethiazide and beta blockers such as propranolol, can affect your blood glucose level. High blood pressure can be difficult

My experience

"When I'm ill, I check my blood glucose every 2–3 hours and do urine tests. If I have ketones, I take more insulin. If I am vomiting, I sip sugary drinks and drink water to flush out ketones." SHELLEY

COMMENT Developing a procedure that you can follow whenever you are unwell will help you stay in control of your diabetes and avoid potential problems. When you have Type 1 diabetes, testing for ketones is particularly important to identify when the illness is becoming serious.

to treat when you have diabetes, so you might need two or three different types of tablets in combination to keep it under control. If the tablets you take affect your blood glucose it is still extremely important to take them, because reducing high blood pressure is just as important as lowering blood glucose in the prevention of long-term complications (see pp.206–208). If you start new medication, monitoring your blood glucose level to assess its effect will tell you whether you need to change your dose or type of tablets or insulin to compensate.

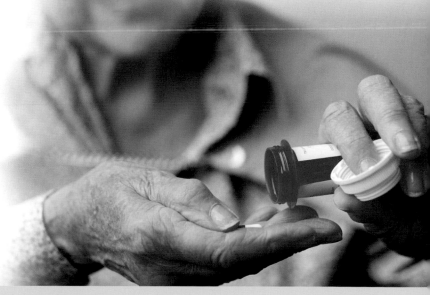

TAKING DIABETES TABLETS
When you are unwell, you should keep taking your diabetes tablets and/or insulin – even if you are not eating – to combat the effect of illness on your blood glucose.

Steroid treatment

Steroids, such as prednisolone or dexamethasone, can have a significant effect on your blood glucose. These are used to reduce inflammation, and to treat a variety of different conditions including:
- Chronic lung conditions: chronic obstructive airways disease, asthma.
- Chronic bowel conditions: Crohn's disease, ulcerative colitis.
- Joint inflammation: rheumatoid arthritis.
- Cancer.

Steroid treatment is also used after organ transplantation to reduce the possibility of rejection. Steroid tablets or injections increase your blood glucose level, and you will need to increase the dose of your tablets or insulin to compensate, even if you are only taking steroids for a short time. Even if you don't have diabetes, steroids can increase your blood glucose level and cause diabetes to develop. Taking steroids via an inhaler or a skin patch will not affect your blood glucose in the same way that tablets and injections do.

Taking a combination of tablets

When you have diabetes, you may find yourself taking five or more different types of tablets and perhaps insulin injections, too, to control not only your blood glucose but also your blood pressure and blood fat levels. If you have other conditions, such as diabetes complications, you may need to take even more.

> **Steroid tablets or injections increase your blood glucose level and you will need to increase the dose of your tablets or insulin to compensate.**

Q I have had tablets for my blood pressure for some time. Now I've been given another type to take as well. I don't feel any different – do I really need to take both?

A Many people need more than one type of tablet for good blood pressure control. Most tablets are prescribed on a trial basis – you need to take them for a while to find out whether they work for you. Although taking lots of tablets may seem like a chore, the treatment you receive is aimed at preventing health problems in the future, so you need to persevere if you are to benefit in the long term.

However many tablets you are prescribed, you should take them all as instructed – even if they don't seem to make a difference to the way you feel. Your treatment is designed to keep you healthy in the long term. If you are concerned about the number of tablets you take, ask your doctor or pharmacist to check regularly that they are all still necessary.

Going into hospital

If you are admitted to hospital, whether as a result of your diabetes – if you develop diabetic ketoacidosis, for example, or you have a diabetes complication – or for something unrelated, such as a broken leg, you will need to make decisions about your diabetes care with hospital staff.

In hospital, your treatment, mealtimes, and blood glucose testing routine will not be the same as at home. To enable your body to recover normally, your blood glucose level should be less than 10 millimoles per litre most of the time. To achieve this, your tablets or insulin should be given at the correct time in relation to your meals, and your usual dose of medication may even need to be increased. If you need snacks between meals or at bedtime, these should be made available, or you might keep some supplies yourself.

You may need to let staff know when you need to test your blood glucose or need your tablets or insulin, as they won't be as familiar with your diabetes as you are. You may be able to do your own tests and take your own medication, or ask for them when you need them. If you are concerned about your diabetes, you need to discuss this with senior staff.

If you are unable to eat or drink for more than a few hours, such as for an operation for which you need an empty stomach, or if you are unconscious, hospital staff will take over your diabetes care. Your blood glucose will be carefully controlled using an insulin infusion and glucose drip, which are inserted into your vein. The rate at which insulin enters your bloodstream is adjusted according to your blood glucose level, which is measured every hour.

As soon as you are eating properly, the glucose drip and insulin infusion will be removed. You can then resume your normal diabetes treatment. Ideally, you will have the first dose of your usual treatment shortly before the drip and infusion are removed to make sure that your blood glucose doesn't rise as a result of the insulin supply suddenly being removed before your usual treatment has had time to work.

When you are discharged

During your hospital stay, changes may have been made to your diabetes tablets or insulin type or regimen. It is important that you know about any new medication, when to take it, and how. If you don't understand why it has changed or what effect it might have, speak to a health professional before you leave. If you have been far less active in hospital than normal and you take insulin-stimulating tablets or insulin, you might be at risk of a hypo when you resume your normal activities, so discuss whether the discharge dose will still be right for you when you get home.

Outpatient visits

If you attend hospital as an outpatient, such as for an investigation or minor operation, you may be asked not to eat or drink for several hours beforehand. If you take insulin-stimulating tablets or insulin, and are unable to balance these with food, you will be at risk of hypoglycaemia. To prevent a hypo, reduce your dose before you begin to fast and test your blood glucose regularly while you are not eating or drinking and during the procedure. If you cannot do your own testing for any reason, staff will need to take over.

When you have diabetes, most procedures take place early in the day so that you can resume your normal treatment as quickly as possible.

Women's health

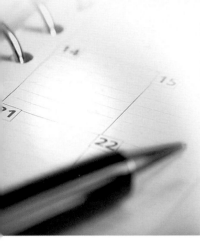

If you are a woman with diabetes, it is important to know how your hormones and common female complaints can affect your blood glucose level. If you plan to have children, it is essential to prepare well before you conceive and to manage your diabetes strictly during pregnancy to safeguard your own and your baby's health and to maximize your chances of a trouble-free labour and delivery. If you develop gestational diabetes, you will need to take similar care to manage this condition.

Practical tips

AVOIDING MENSTRUAL HIGHS AND LOWS

- Try to stick to your healthy eating plan, even if you feel like eating less healthy foods.
- Limit your salt intake, as this causes water retention.
- Cut back on alcohol, caffeine, and chocolate – these can affect your blood glucose level as well as your mood.
- Eat at regular intervals to avoid swings in your blood glucose level.
- Do some regular physical activity – you may find that being active improves your mood and makes it easier to control your blood glucose level.

Female hormones

The female hormones oestrogen and progesterone are produced by the ovaries. Together, these hormones regulate your menstrual cycle and maintain a pregnancy.

Your menstrual cycle

During your menstrual cycle, levels of oestrogen and progesterone in your body rise and fall. At the beginning of your cycle, oestrogen causes the lining of the uterus to thicken. If conception does not occur, more progesterone is produced to trigger the shedding of the uterine lining. You may find that these monthly hormonal fluctuations have an effect on your blood glucose level.

If you suspect that your menstrual cycle is affecting your blood glucose, testing your blood glucose level frequently (four or more times a day) just before, during, and directly after your period and recording the results will help you to identify any regular pattern. If you find that your blood glucose level tends to rise just before your period, you could:
- Try fitting in some extra physical activity to bring your blood glucose level down.
- Avoid eating too many extra carbohydrates.
- Try increasing your insulin dose in the few days before your period is due.

If, on the other hand, your blood glucose is lower than normal and you have a tendency to have more hypos, you could:
- Try increasing your intake of carbohydrate-containing foods.
- Reduce your insulin dose in the few days before your period.

The way in which your periods affect your blood glucose is likely to remain fairly constant – so even if you change your diabetes

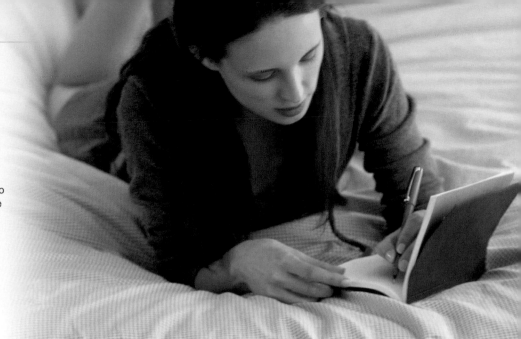

treatment, over time you should be able to work out how to keep your blood glucose balanced throughout your monthly cycle.

Menopause

Many changes occur in a woman's body during the menopause, but these will not necessarily affect your diabetes and its treatment. However, you may find that some symptoms of the menopause are similar to those that occur when you have a high or low blood glucose level. If you do feel hot, shaky, or start sweating, testing your blood glucose level can help you decide whether you need to treat your diabetes at this time.

You may wish to consider hormone replacement therapy (HRT), which relieves menopausal symptoms. Ask your health professional whether taking HRT would be right for you.

Cystitis and thrush

Inflammation of the bladder lining, which is known as cystitis, and a fungal infection of the vagina, known as thrush, are conditions that commonly affect women. Cystitis is generally caused by a bacterial infection and causes frequent and painful passing of urine. Thrush develops when a fungus called *Candida albicans*, which can occur naturally in the vagina, grows more rapidly than usual. Thrush can cause unpleasant itching and a discharge. Cystitis and thrush can occur more frequently when you have diabetes because a slightly raised blood glucose level provides the type of environment in which bacteria and fungi thrive. An infection can cause your blood glucose level to rise even further (see p.131). If you think you may have cystitis or thrush, see your doctor. Treatment for each of these conditions is available from your doctor or pharmacist.

> Cystitis and thrush can occur more frequently when you have diabetes because a slightly raised blood glucose level provides the type of environment in which bacteria and fungi thrive.

Practical tips

GIVING YOUR BABY THE BEST START

- As for any woman wishing to conceive, you should take a daily dose of folic acid for 3 months before you conceive and during the first 4 months of pregnancy. This improves cell growth and helps to guard against spina bifida and other rare spinal cord defects in your baby.

- Avoid eating pâté, raw shellfish, foods that contain raw eggs, and unpasteurized food, such as certain types of soft or blue-veined cheese, as these may cause infections that can harm your baby.

- Cut out alcohol and cigarettes, and cut down on caffeine.

Pregnancy

Careful planning is very important when it comes to pregnancy and diabetes. Looking after your diabetes all the way through your pregnancy, and attending antenatal appointments will also maximize your chances of having a healthy baby and as few problems as possible. Unless you have gestational diabetes (see pp.144–145), your diabetes will affect your pregnancy (and vice versa) right from the start.

Planning your pregnancy

Having diabetes doesn't make it more or less likely that you will be able to become pregnant, but it does increase the risk of you and your baby having problems. A high blood glucose level, that is an HbA1c level above 7 per cent (see pp.66–67), around the time you conceive and in the first eight weeks of pregnancy, can affect your baby's development. This is why it is so important to plan your pregnancy carefully so that you know that your diabetes is under control when you conceive, and avoid accidental pregnancy by using a reliable method of contraception (see p.127).

If you want to have a baby, your health professional will be able to advise you on your blood glucose control, perform blood tests, check your health in general, and make any necessary referrals. In particular, you will need to have your eyes checked for diabetic retinopathy (see pp.190–194) because, if left untreated, this can worsen during pregnancy.

Before you conceive, you will need to check your blood glucose level at least three to four times a day and make sure that the majority of your tests are in the range of 4–7 millimoles per litre. You may need to work towards this by adjusting your insulin, tablets, food intake, and activity level. You may need to adjust your insulin dose to bring your blood glucose level under tight control. If this is difficult, or causes lots of hypos, you may need to change your insulin regimen – for example, from twice-daily injections to a four-times-a-day regimen. More frequent injections will enable you to fit your insulin dose to your glucose level more accurately. See pp.90–95 for information on adjusting insulin doses and regimens.

If you take tablets to control your diabetes, you may need to take insulin injections instead to achieve the control you need before becoming pregnant. When you do become pregnant you will certainly need to switch to insulin, because tablets for diabetes may be harmful to your baby. You should be able to revert to your tablets once your baby is born if they continue to control your blood glucose. If you start taking insulin, temporarily or permanently, you will need to inform the driving authorities (see p.121).

Once you have your blood glucose well controlled, your HbA1c level should be checked to confirm that it is 7 per cent or less,

ROUTINE ANTENATAL TESTS

Antenatal care starts as soon as you know that you are pregnant and is essential to ensure that the pregnancy is progressing well and that your diabetes is as well controlled as possible. You will have several routine tests at regular intervals throughout your pregnancy.

TEST	WHEN	REASON
HbA1c	Every 1–2 months	To check that your blood glucose level is tightly controlled, to ensure your baby can grow and develop normally.
Retinal examination	Start of pregnancy, then every 3 months	To look for signs of diabetic retinopathy (see pp.192–193), which can develop or worsen during pregnancy.
Ultrasound scan	Every 1–2 months	To assess the development and growth of your baby and detect any abnormalities, using an image produced by sound waves.
Blood pressure	Every visit	To check for raised blood pressure, which increases the risk of pre-eclampsia (p.142).
Urine test	Every visit	To check for the presence of ketones, which can harm your baby.
Fetal monitoring	Every visit	To check your baby's heartbeat and movements.
Blood test for neural tube defects	At 16–18 weeks	To detect severe neural tube defects in your baby, which can cause disorders including spina bifida.
Amniocentesis	(Optional) at 18 weeks	To test for genetic abnormalities.

If your blood glucose level is high, your baby's will be, too. This is because glucose can cross your placenta into your baby's bloodstream – but insulin cannot.

so that when you conceive, your baby will have the best chance of growing and developing normally.

ACE inhibitor tablets for controlling blood pressure, such as lisinopril and ramipril, cannot be taken during pregnancy. Your health professional will be able to suggest alternatives.

While you are pregnant

Good diabetes control is crucial while you are pregnant, both for your baby's and your own health.

If your blood glucose level is high, your baby's will be, too. This is because glucose can cross your placenta into your baby's bloodstream – but insulin cannot. If your baby's glucose level is high, he or she will have to produce more insulin to lower it, which in turn causes extra glucose to be stored in your baby's body, causing faster than normal growth. As a result, you are more likely to experience a difficult labour and delivery and

DEALING WITH HYPOS DURING PREGNANCY

- Eat carbohydrate-containing foods regularly throughout the day.
- Test your blood glucose level at least 4 times a day and adjust your insulin according to the results.
- Sometimes the symptoms of hypoglycaemia change during pregnancy, so if you have an unusual symptom, check your blood glucose straight away – it could be a sign that you are hypo.
- Keep glucose tablets, a glucose drink, or dextrose gel with you at all times to use as soon as you feel hypo symptoms coming on.
- Tell your partner, a friend, or a work colleague that hypoglycaemia could occur, and if possible, show him or her how to give you a glucagon injection (see p.109), should you become unconscious.

your baby may have problems with breathing and could experience hypoglycaemia after birth.

If you have Type 1 diabetes, another reason to keep your blood glucose level regulated during pregnancy is to prevent ketones from forming (see p.113). Ketones can be extremely harmful to your baby and, in rare situations, can even be fatal to your baby. Ketones can form during pregnancy even if your blood glucose level is not high enough to give you symptoms, so it is vital that you increase your insulin dose as soon as your blood glucose level starts to rise.

Throughout your pregnancy, you need to keep your pre-meal blood glucose level between 4–6 millimoles per litre and, 2 hours after meals, at 4–7 millimoles per litre. You should also keep your HbA1c at 7 per cent or below.

As your pregnancy progresses, you will need larger doses of insulin to keep your blood glucose well controlled. This is because your growing baby and the additional hormones your placenta produces increase your body's need for insulin. By the ninth month, your original dose of insulin may have doubled, trebled, or more. As soon as your baby is born, your body's insulin requirement will reduce and you will revert to a dose close to what you were taking before you became pregnant.

■ **MORNING SICKNESS** In the early weeks of pregnancy, you may feel nauseous at any time. If you feel sick in the morning, try having a drink or a plain

biscuit before you get up, and split your morning dose of insulin so that you take some when you normally would and the rest later when you feel like eating. To combat queasiness at other times, eat regular snacks of plain biscuits, crackers, or fruit.

If you are vomiting and can't keep food down, your health professional can prescribe pregnancy-safe medicines that prevent sickness and give you advice on your insulin regimen. If you are extremely unwell and there is a danger that your body might be producing ketones, you may be admitted to hospital for treatment.

■ **ANTENATAL CARE** Your antenatal care is especially important when you have diabetes. You will need to attend an antenatal clinic at least once a fortnight right from the start of your pregnancy, at which both obstetric and diabetes health professionals should be present. You will be offered a diabetes and antenatal record book, with details of who to contact between appointments if you need to.

At the clinic, you will be able to discuss the results of your home tests and any problems you are having. For example, you may experience more frequent, sudden, and severe episodes of hypoglycaemia, especially in the first three months of your pregnancy, when your body's need for insulin can fluctuate unpredictably.

■ **LOOKING AFTER YOURSELF** Eating healthily, being physically active on a regular basis – a brisk daily walk, gentle jog (if you are used to it), or swimming – and avoiding alcohol and cigarettes will all increase your chances of a successful, comfortable pregnancy. You should not attempt to diet when you are pregnant because you need enough energy for both you and your baby.

If you become unwell for any reason during your pregnancy, your blood glucose level will rise and you will need more insulin. You should monitor your blood glucose level as you would normally, and correct it with insulin as necessary (see p.94). You should also test your urine or blood for ketones twice a day, and contact your health professional straight away if ketones are present.

Very occasionally, babies die during the last few weeks of pregnancy. This is a more common occurrence when you have diabetes, but is still very rare. The chances of it happening to you are reduced if your diabetes has

My experience

"I would say that someone with diabetes receives even better antenatal care than someone who doesn't have it – so just for once, diabetes has its perks!" LOUISE

COMMENT Although you need more frequent clinic visits when you are pregnant, you tend to see the same people each time and have very detailed tests and attention – so it can make you feel extra special.

been very well controlled. If there is a risk to your baby, you may be offered an induction or Caesarean section before your expected birth date.

■ **PLANNING THE BIRTH** Because you may need special care during labour, you will probably be advised to have your baby in hospital rather than at home. Talk to your health professional in advance to find out the options that are available in your area and what you can expect to happen to you and your baby during the birth.

KEEPING ACTIVE
Regular physical activity helps to prepare you for the physical demands of labour and speed recovery after the birth. Swimming is a particularly comfortable form of exercise when you are pregnant because your weight is supported by the water.

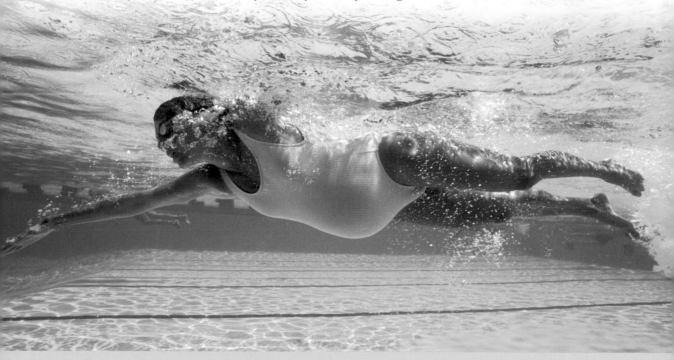

Giving birth

Your labour may start normally, if all has gone well with your pregnancy, or you may need to be induced or have a Caesarean section if problems have arisen. If labour is progressing normally, you may wish to monitor your own blood glucose level, or ask your partner to do it for you. You need to test at least once an hour to monitor the level. If you have been advised not to eat (in case you should need an emergency general anaesthetic), you are more likely to have a hypo, so regular blood glucose testing will warn you of this. Make sure that you give all your test results to hospital staff for their records.

If labour lasts a long time or starts when your glucose level may be falling, such as when you have not eaten for some time, you will probably be given an intravenous glucose drip

Once your baby is separated from your placenta, his or her blood glucose level falls. For this reason, when your baby is born, a blood sample will be taken to check whether he or she is hypoglycaemic.

POTENTIAL PREGNANCY PROBLEMS

Most pregnancies progress smoothly, but all pregnant women face potential problems. Having diabetes makes some problems more likely. Healthy eating, regular physical activity, and excellent blood glucose control all greatly reduce the risk of difficulties occurring.

PROBLEM	IMPLICATIONS
Worsening of diabetes complications	If you already have eye complications, they may worsen in pregnancy. Your eyes are checked as part of your antenatal care so that any problems can be treated early. Kidney problems before pregnancy can increase your risk of raised blood pressure, so this is also checked regularly.
Oversized baby	A high blood glucose level can cause your baby to grow at an increased rate (known as macrosomia). Excellent blood glucose control reduces the risk of macrosomia. If it occurs, your baby may need to be delivered early.
Polyhydramnios	If your baby has a high blood glucose level, he or she may produce more urine, which can lead to an excessive amount of amniotic fluid in the uterus. Polyhydramnios can cause premature labour.
Pre-eclampsia	If severe or left untreated, pre-eclampsia can lead to a potentially fatal disorder known as eclampsia that causes seizures and may bring on a coma. If you have high blood pressure, protein in your urine, and fluid retention in the last 3 months of pregnancy, you are likely to be monitored in hospital until your baby is born, or if you are near your delivery date, labour may be induced.
Premature labour	If labour starts before the 37th week of pregnancy, or you are induced early, your baby may not be fully developed and may need special care when he or she is born.

to keep your blood glucose stable until your baby is born. You will also receive an infusion of insulin via a vein, and the amounts will be adjusted according to your blood glucose level (see p.135). Your baby's heart rate, movements, and position will be checked throughout your labour. You can expect to be offered the same pain relief choices as any other mother, depending on how your labour is progressing.

After your baby is born

Once your baby is separated from your placenta, his or her blood glucose level falls. For this reason, when your baby is born, a blood sample will be taken to check whether he or she is hypoglycaemic. If your baby has been born early but is the right size for a full-term pregnancy, there is a danger that his or her lungs may not be fully developed. As a result, your baby's breathing will also be carefully checked and, if necessary, he or she will be helped to breathe at first.

If all is well, you should be able to feed your baby immediately, although he or she may also need a glucose injection or bottle feed to increase a low blood glucose level. If your baby

is seriously hypoglycaemic or is having difficulty breathing, he or she may be moved to a special care baby unit to be closely monitored. In some hospitals, babies born to mothers with diabetes are routinely taken to a special care unit for observation immediately after birth.

After the delivery of your placenta, your need for insulin reduces suddenly and if you were receiving an insulin infusion during labour, the dosage rate will be lowered immediately to prevent you from becoming hypoglycaemic. Unless you have had a general anaesthetic, you will be able to eat and drink soon after the birth. You should then be able to take over your blood glucose testing

Myth OR TRUTH?

MYTH
If you have diabetes, your baby will be born with diabetes.

TRUTH
Babies are rarely born with diabetes. Your child will have an increased risk of developing either Type 1 or Type 2 diabetes (depending on the type you have or your family history), but the risk is for their lifetime, and not at the time of birth.

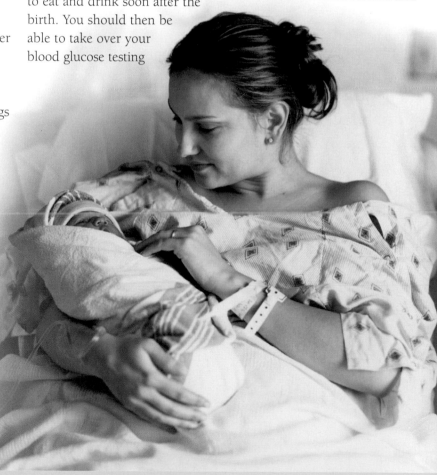

A growing baby and the hormones your body produces increase the demand for insulin, and if your body is unable to meet this need your blood glucose level will rise.

and insulin injections. You may be able to revert to tablets if you were taking these before you were pregnant, unless you are breastfeeding. You cannot take tablets for diabetes when you are breastfeeding, because they will affect your baby via your milk. You may need to continue taking insulin until you wean your baby.

If you weren't taking insulin or tablets before you became pregnant, you may be able to revert to controlling your blood glucose through healthy eating and physical activity, in which case there are no special considerations with regard to breastfeeding.

Gestational diabetes

It is not possible to determine whether you are susceptible to gestational diabetes before your first pregnancy until the condition becomes apparent – which is most likely to happen at about 28 weeks.

A growing baby and the hormones your body produces increase the demand for insulin, and if your body is unable to meet this need, your blood glucose level will rise above

normal. You will need a laboratory blood test to diagnose gestational diabetes, and specialist antenatal care if you are found to have the condition.

Gestational diabetes usually disappears once your baby is born, but occasionally you may develop permanent Type 1 or Type 2 diabetes while you are pregnant. If you develop gestational diabetes, you have an increased risk of gestational diabetes in future pregnancies and of developing permanent Type 2 diabetes in later years. You can reduce the likelihood of this happening by taking regular physical activity and keeping your weight in the recommended range (see p.46).

Diagnosis and treatment

The first sign of gestational diabetes is often a positive urine test for glucose. However, because it is common for pregnant women to have glucose in their urine, you will need to have one of two laboratory blood tests – a fasting or a random blood glucose test or an oral glucose tolerance test (see pp.20–21) to confirm your diagnosis. If you are diagnosed with gestational diabetes, you will receive the same antenatal care as any other woman with diabetes who is pregnant, to limit the risks to yourself and your baby (see pp.139–140).

Depending on your blood glucose level at diagnosis and the stage of your pregnancy, your initial treatment may involve adjusting your food intake. If you have been eating a lot of high-sugar foods, large meals containing lots of carbohydrate, or having sugary drinks, limiting these can make a big difference immediately to your blood glucose level. You should aim to keep your pre-meal blood glucose level between 4–6 millimoles per litre and 2 hours after meals at 4–7 millimoles per litre. Your health professional will show you how to test your own blood glucose level (see pp.62–75) to reveal how effective any changes to your eating habits have been.

If healthier eating is not enough to keep your blood glucose level in the recommended range, you will be offered insulin injections. Tablets used to treat diabetes cannot be taken during pregnancy because there is a risk that they may harm your baby, whereas insulin is perfectly safe to use. You may need up to four injections each day to maintain tight control of your blood glucose level.

Birth and postnatal care
Because there is a possibility that your baby will need to be delivered by Caesarean section or require care in a special unit once he or she is born, you will probably be advised to have your baby in hospital. During labour, you may also need a glucose drip and an insulin infusion (see p.135) and more frequent monitoring of your blood pressure and your baby's movements and progress.

As soon as your baby is born, your body's need for insulin will reduce dramatically, so you will probably no longer require insulin treatment or need to check your blood glucose level. However, because there is a small risk of developing permanent Type 1 or Type 2 diabetes when you are pregnant, you will either have a continuing need for insulin treatment or have an oral glucose tolerance test six weeks after the birth of your baby to check that your body is still able to use glucose properly. For this reason, you may wish to continue to check your blood glucose level yourself for the few weeks before your formal glucose test. Whatever you do, you should be aware of diabetes-related symptoms (see pp.18–19) and see your health professional as soon as possible if you experience any of them.

Once you have had gestational diabetes, it is likely to recur in future pregnancies. You are also much more likely to develop Type 2 diabetes later in life. If you are overweight, if other family members have Type 2 diabetes, or if your family comes from South Asia, Africa, or the Caribbean, your risk is even greater. Once you have had gestational diabetes, you will need a fasting blood glucose test or oral glucose tolerance test at least every three years to check for Type 2 diabetes.

You can delay or even prevent the onset of Type 2 diabetes by keeping your weight in the recommended range for your height, taking regular physical activity, and eating healthily. If you experience any symptoms of diabetes, see your health professional.

Myth OR TRUTH?

MYTH
You cannot breastfeed if you have diabetes.

TRUTH Breastfeeding is an ideal start for your baby and having diabetes doesn't make it any less likely that you and your baby will be successful in this. You cannot take tablets to control diabetes while you are breastfeeding, but there are other ways of managing your diabetes if you wish to breastfeed. Your health professional can advise you.

Life with a new baby

For any family, adjusting to life with a new baby can take time. Meals, sleep, and time to yourself or with your partner are all likely to be disrupted, which means that your diabetes routine will also be upset.

Although you can be a little less strict about your blood glucose control now that you are no longer pregnant, there are aspects of motherhood, such as breastfeeding, that may make a difference to your diabetes. Knowing what to expect as a new mother and how to manage your diabetes in these situations will help you through this period of adjustment.

Eating and drinking

Your mealtimes are likely to be irregular when you have a new baby, and this can affect your diabetes. If you go without food for too long and you take insulin or insulin-stimulating tablets, you can become hypoglycaemic or, if there are extended periods of time between your insulin doses, your blood glucose level may rise. You may find it useful to prepare or set aside some sandwiches, fruit, or cereal bars each day in case you are unable to eat or drink when planned. If your mealtimes are unpredictable and you take a ready-mixed insulin or are on a twice-a-day regimen, changing to a more flexible four-times-a-day system might suit your new lifestyle better.

Breastfeeding

When you breastfeed, you transfer energy to your baby through your milk. This means that you will need to eat at least an additional 50g of carbohydrate per day (see pp.35–36). If you take insulin, you may also need to reduce your dose to prevent hypoglycaemia.

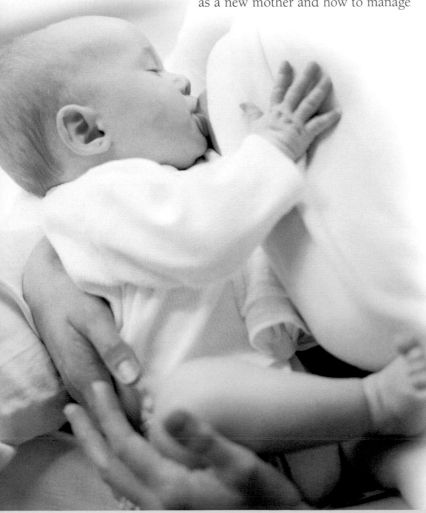

BREASTFEEDING
Breastfeeding is as suitable for your baby as for any other, and you have just the same chances of success as any other mother. If you take insulin, you may need to reduce your dose while you are breastfeeding, to prevent hypoglycaemia.

When you are feeding, keep your hypo treatments or snacks to hand. Like other breastfeeding mothers, you will probably find that you need to drink more sugar-free fluid than normal to prevent dehydration.

Sleeping

If you sleep when your baby sleeps, you will probably be "cat-napping" throughout the day. Unfortunately, this can result in a hypo if you doze when you are due to eat a meal, or hyperglycaemia if you sleep late and miss your injection time because you were awake most of the night. You may need to consider how to adapt your insulin regimen if an unpredictable sleeping pattern is causing serious swings in your blood glucose level.

Coping with stress

Looking after your new baby and trying to keep good control of your diabetes can be very stressful.

Q I'm really worried that I might have a hypo when I'm alone with my baby. How can I make sure that this doesn't happen?

A In order to guard against hypos, test your blood glucose level frequently. Keep glucose tablets or glucose drinks in any room you might be using and if you feel a hypo coming on, treat it straight away, whether or not you can test your blood glucose level. Eat regularly, and have a snack if you get up to feed your baby at night. Don't nap or sleep on an empty stomach and try not to put your baby's feeds before your own food needs.

After working so hard to manage your blood glucose during pregnancy, it can be difficult to relax that very tight control and allow yourself to start aiming for good control again. You may even feel guilty if your blood glucose level is within the ideal range less often than it was when you were pregnant. Finding time to test, eat, and inject as you would like may also be a strain.

It is also very common for new mothers to feel low or miserable during the first few days or weeks after childbirth. Having diabetes won't make you any more or less likely to experience this mood change, known as the "baby blues", nor more serious post-natal depression. However, feeling like this can affect your energy levels and your ability to manage your diabetes as well as your new baby's needs.

If you feel that you are not coping as well as you would like, you may find it helpful to talk to your health professional about different ways of dealing with motherhood and diabetes.

For everyday times when you are feeling low, simply talking to your health professional or family or friends can be helpful. Taking exercise when you can fit it in can be a useful way of relieving stress and meeting other people in a similar position to yourself. If you experience ongoing depression, you may need treatment (see pp.186–189). The more options you have for dealing with stressful times, the better you will be able to cope when they occur.

Myth OR TRUTH?

MYTH
You don't need to worry about your diabetes control once you've had your baby.

TRUTH
The tight control needed during pregnancy means keeping your pre-meal blood glucose level at 4–6 millimoles per litre, and two hours after a meal at 4–7 millimoles per litre. When you have had your baby, a blood glucose level that is higher than this, even for a day or two, is less likely to do harm, although your overall aim should still be to keep your level in the range of 4–7 millimoles per litre. This will keep you well in the long term and reduce your risk of developing complications in future.

Benefiting from health care

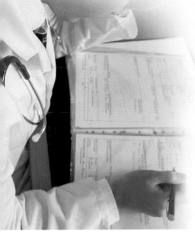

Having diabetes means that you probably use health care services more often than someone who doesn't have the condition. Regular health checks are a routine part of your life, and you may need extra help if you are having difficulties with your diabetes management. Your health professional plays an important role in keeping you well, but the more knowledgeable you are about your diabetes and the more input you have, the better controlled your diabetes is likely to be.

Keeping yourself informed

To get the most from the health care you receive, you need to be informed about your own diabetes. The more you know about your condition, the more in control of your diabetes you can be. Your health professionals will help and support you, but it's you who bears the greatest responsibility for your day-to-day diabetes care. Ask yourself the following questions to identify any gaps in your knowledge. If you are unsure of the facts, make a list of the questions you cannot answer so that you can ask them at your next appointment.

■ **WHAT TYPE OF DIABETES DO YOU HAVE?** This information is vital to enable you to understand your treatment and look after yourself properly. The type of diabetes you have always remains the same (unless you have gestational diabetes, see pp.144–145) even if

your treatment changes over time. For example, if you have Type 2 diabetes and start insulin treatment, you still have Type 2 diabetes.

■ **WHAT TARGETS ARE YOU AND YOUR HEALTH PROFESSIONAL AIMING FOR?** Targets given throughout this book are a general guide for everyone, but there may be specific HbA1c levels, home monitoring results, or blood pressure levels that you and your health professional want to achieve. If your diabetes has been out of control for a while, for example, it will probably take time to improve your levels and your targets might change from one appointment to the next. Knowing what your targets are will help you work with your health professional to achieve them.

■ **WHAT TREATMENT ARE YOU TAKING FOR YOUR DIABETES?** Knowing the names of your tablets or insulin is helpful, particularly if you attend appointments

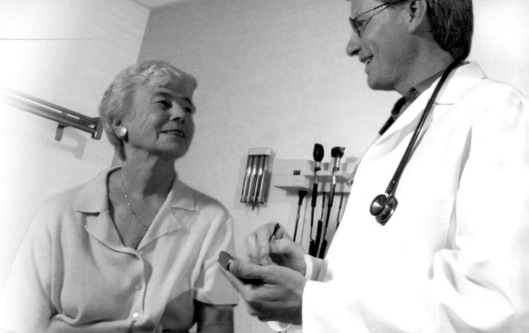

REVIEWING YOUR CARE
The treatment you receive for your diabetes will keep changing throughout your life to reflect changes in your body and your lifestyle. Your health professionals will work with you to continually review your care.

with health professionals who do not know you very well. Part of your responsibility is to take your medication at the right times, such as in relation to meals, so that it is as effective as possible. It is also very important to take your treatment regularly, every day.

■ **ARE YOU DEVELOPING ANY LONG-TERM COMPLICATIONS OF DIABETES?** When you have your health checks, you should be told what the results are.

> **Q** How often do I need to make an appointment to see my health professional – is it only once a year at my annual review?

> **A** Aside from your annual review, additional appointments depend on specific aspects of your diabetes care. For example, if any of your tablets change, you will need to see your health professional within about 3 months to assess whether this has helped. More urgent problems, such as foot ulcers, may mean you are seen twice a week.

So you should know if there are any changes in your eyes, kidneys, feet, or heart, what changes to look for, and in what situations you should ask to be seen urgently.

■ **ARE THERE ANY OTHER HEALTH PROBLEMS CONNECTED TO YOUR DIABETES?** Diabetes is a complex disease that can affect other aspects of your health (or vice versa). If you are unsure whether other health problems, for example stomach upsets or aches and pains, are related to your diabetes, you should clarify this at your next appointment, and make sure you understand the answers you are given.

Getting the most from your appointments

You will probably develop a regular relationship with one or two people, and see other health professionals occasionally. You may have all your health checks carried out by different

Your health care professionals will help and support you, but it's you who bears the greatest responsibility for your day-to-day diabetes care.

My experience

"The health professionals I have seen have given me helpful advice. They are always prepared to listen to my worries and fears, however irrational these seem to be." SHELLEY

COMMENT It's very important to have open conversations with health professionals so that they can help you to deal with your diabetes. If you don't voice your concerns, you may find it difficult to address them on your own. The expertise offered by your health professional can be invaluable – so don't hesitate to make the best use of it.

to see someone who is specifically trained to treat and monitor those problems and provide you with more specific advice.

Preparing for your annual review

Your annual diabetes review is a two-way consultation between you and your health professional. Although you may have other appointments outside of the annual review, this yearly overview is an important part of your diabetes care. You have the opportunity to ask questions about your diabetes and discuss anything that is concerning you. Your health professional needs to know how you've been managing your diabetes so that he or she can assess whether any changes are necessary and help you with any concerns.

people or by one individual, depending on how services are organized in your area. Routine tests (such as having your eyes photographed or your feet examined) can be carried out by any health professional trained to perform that test. However, if you start to develop problems (with your eyes or feet, for example), you should expect

MONITORING YOUR HEALTH
During your annual review, your health professional will perform a number of tests, including checking your blood pressure, to assess your overall health.

It's important to prepare for your appointment so that you can give your health professional as much information as possible and work together to decide on the best course of action. Before your appointment, write down any of the following:

- A regularly fluctuating blood glucose level.
- Side effects to medication.
- Changes you have made to your insulin or medication.
- Problems with equipment.
- Questions about new equipment or treatment.
- Lifestyle changes you have made or are planning, such as a new job or travel plans.

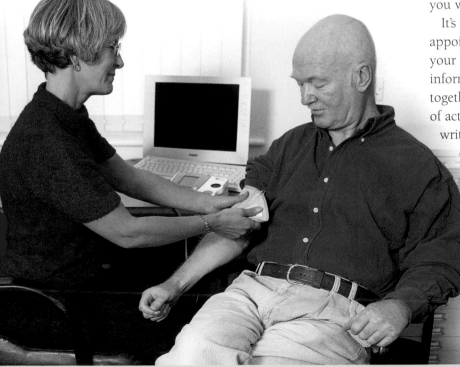

- If you are planning a pregnancy.
- Any difficulties with coping or keeping up your diabetes care.

During your annual review

As part of your annual review, your health professional will do the following or arrange for it to be done:
- Perform an HbA1c test to measure your long-term blood glucose level (see pp.66–67).
- Perform blood and urine tests to check kidney function and blood fat levels.
- Check your weight and body mass index (BMI).
- Examine your legs and feet to check your skin, circulation, and nerve supply.
- Check your blood pressure.
- Examine your eyes.
- Examine your injection sites if you are taking insulin.

If any problems are found, you will be referred for the appropriate treatment. You should feel free to talk about how you are coping with your diabetes at home, work, school, or college, and to raise any issues you might be concerned about, such as stress, physical activity, healthy eating, smoking or alcohol consumption, and sexual problems.

If, at any time, you don't understand what is being said, or you are unclear about any terms used, ask for an explanation. You can also discuss with your health professional the timing of your next appointment. You may wish to give yourself some time to try a new treatment or lifestyle change in order to see the benefits, or you may prefer to return to the clinic earlier if you feel you need some support in making any changes.

After your annual review

If you need to make any changes to your diabetes care, you should know why these changes need to be made, what effects they will have, and what to do if the changes do not produce the desired result. If you are asked to attend any other clinic appointment, check that you understand why it is necessary. It's a good idea to write down important information – after a long discussion you may not be able to remember everything that has been said.

To ensure that you leave your review with all the knowledge you need, make a note of the following:
- How your diabetes is and whether there are any concerns about your present or future health.
- Changes (if any) you need to make to your tablets or insulin, including how often you take your medication and at what times of the day.
- What effect any change in treatment will have – how quickly it will work, how much it will affect your blood glucose level, what side effects you should look out for, and what action to take should they occur.
- Any additional treatment or appointments you need.
- Who to contact (and how) if you need help or advice before your next appointment.

Practical tips

CONTACTING YOUR HEALTH PROFESSIONAL

You should contact your health professional between appointments if you are experiencing any of the following:
- Frequent or severe low blood glucose levels.
- A consistently high blood glucose level.
- Injuries to your feet that are not healing.
- Sudden changes in your vision.
- Problems with medication or equipment.
- Feeling unable to cope.

If, at any time, you don't understand what is being said, or you are unclear about any terms used, ask for an explanation.

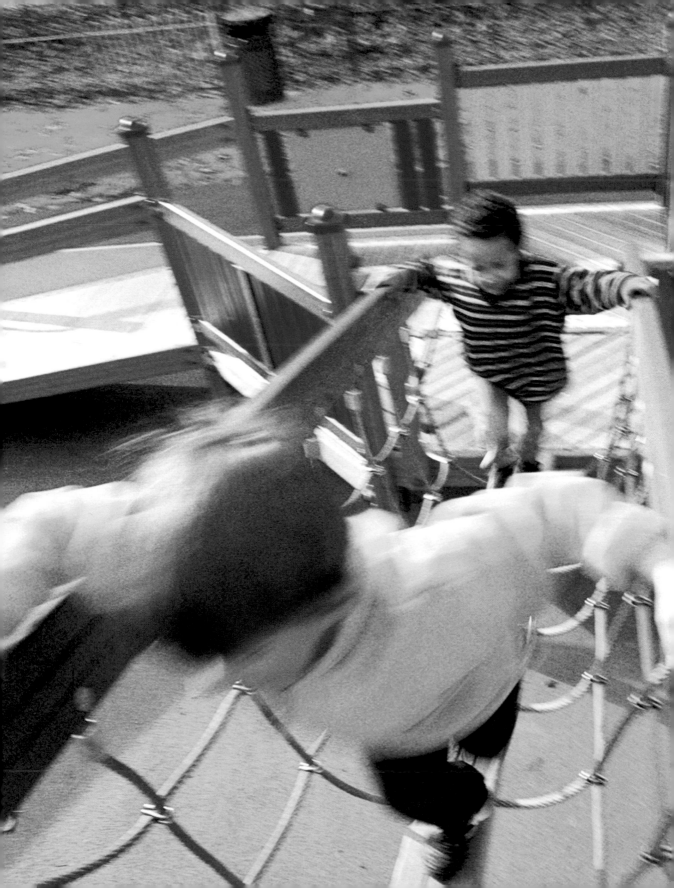

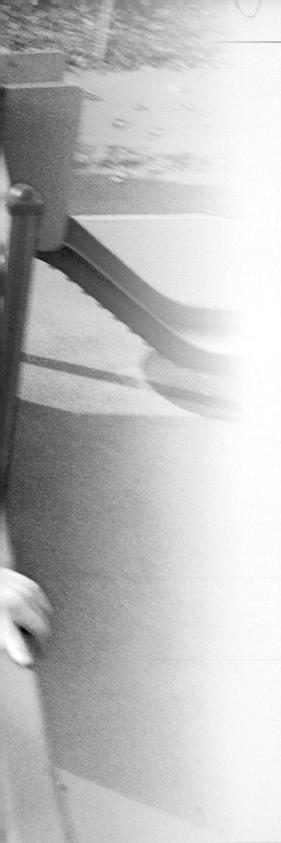

Children and teenagers

Diabetes can develop in babies or toddlers, later during childhood, during the teenage years, or beyond. Although age does not affect the type of treatment, diabetes care can be tailored to a child's needs at each stage of his or her development.

As a parent of a young child with diabetes, you bear the greatest responsibility for managing the condition. You need to inform carers; make sure your child is able to eat at the right time; monitor his or her blood glucose level and act on the results; inject insulin; and deal with hypos.

As a parent of a school-age child with diabetes, you need to liaise with teachers closely. Increasingly, your child will come to understand the importance of good blood glucose control and preventing hypos, and you can work together to achieve this.

Teenagers and young adults are able to care more for their own diabetes with support from parents. As a teenager, you may feel that your diabetes sometimes restricts your freedom. By becoming adept at integrating diabetes into your lifestyle, however, you can manage it successfully, and still live your life to the full.

Babies and young children

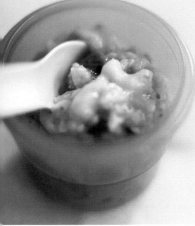

Caring for a baby or young child with diabetes places many demands on you as a parent. You need to give insulin injections, perform blood tests, and make sure that your child eats foods that have a beneficial effect on his or her diabetes. You also need to know how to act at times when your child is reluctant to let you do these things, what to do when his or her blood glucose level is too low, and how to care for your child when he or she is unwell.

Diabetes, your child, and you

It is rare for children under five to develop diabetes, but Type 1 diabetes can occur in babies when they are only a few months old (Type 2 diabetes never occurs in children under five). The symptoms of diabetes, such as passing a lot of urine and being very thirsty, are the same in children under five as in adults (see pp.18–19). Symptoms can become apparent very quickly – over a few days or a week – you might have noticed that your child's nappy needed changing more often, or that he or she started to wet the bed, or needed extra feeds and drinks.

Discovering that your young child has diabetes can give rise to many emotions: you may feel angry, upset, guilty, helpless, or anxious, and you may worry whether you will be able to cope with the level of care your

child will need every day. Because your child is so young, you will have the responsibility for looking after his or diabetes, which can make your job as a parent even more demanding. Your young child with diabetes needs food at regular intervals, blood tests, and insulin injections. Your child might not yet be able to tell you how he or she feels, so making sure that his or her blood glucose does not fall to a level at which hypoglycaemia (see pp.102–109) can occur is also your responsibility.

However, you are not alone. You have the full support of diabetes health professionals as you learn more about diabetes and what you need to do to take care of your child.

It is important to take your child to diabetes clinics and you will be visited by diabetes health professionals on a regular basis to discuss your child's growth and

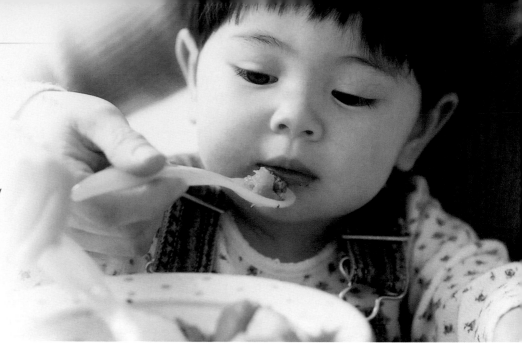

REGULAR EATING
Encouraging your child to eat regular meals and snacks containing complex carbohydrates is particularly important when he or she has diabetes.

development, and diabetes control. Keeping your child's blood glucose level between 4–7 millimoles per litre helps to reduce the risk of complications when he or she is older.

Telling other people

Your family and friends will probably be concerned about your child's diabetes and they will almost certainly want to know more about it. In general, it's up to you to decide how much to say and to whom, but you will need to give more detailed information to people who care for your child, such as nursery school staff, babysitters, or childminders.

When you tell people that your young child has diabetes, you will probably find that they respond in a variety of ways. People who are close to you may be upset and unsure how to treat your child. You may find it difficult to support and reassure others when it is all new to you, too,

but it is important to try to help people understand what you are going through and to appreciate how they are feeling too. If you have other children, they should also feel included in what is happening.

Whoever you talk to, you will probably find that everyone has something to say about diabetes, regardless of whether it is relevant to you and your child. When dealing with other people's reactions, you might want to prepare yourself with some stock answers to common

My experience

"Sometimes our daughter feels jealous of the attention her brother gets ... it hasn't been easy. When she tries to get involved with his diabetes it usually ends in fighting!" VICKY

COMMENT Siblings of children with diabetes can sometimes feel left out. They may start to behave differently in an effort to get more of your attention. If this happens, you may need to spend time alone with them so that they feel "special" too.

As your child grows, he or she will need to eat enough carbohydrate at mealtimes and throughout the day to keep his or her blood glucose level in the recommended range.

questions such as "What's diabetes?" "How did he or she get it?", or "Will he or she grow out of it?". If people try to give you advice, you could answer, "Thank you, I'll think about that", or "I've been told diabetes is very individual". You may sometimes receive conflicting advice from other people or health professionals – talk this through with your diabetes health professional to see how it relates specifically to your child's diabetes.

■ **TALKING TO CARERS** You need to make sure that anyone who looks after your child is given enough information about your child's diabetes, for example:

- What diabetes means.
- Your child's eating and drinking requirements.
- What treatments and blood glucose tests your child needs and when.
- Symptoms that might suggest hyperglycaemia.
- Symptoms that might suggest hypoglycaemia.
- What to do if your child has a hypo.
- What to do if your child is unwell.
- Your contact details at all times.
- Your GP's contact details.

Your child's carer will probably want to ask lots of questions and is likely to be worried or even frightened about giving injections or testing your child's blood. Reassure him or her by demonstrating exactly what is involved. You may need to repeat the information regularly before it becomes familiar to your child's carer.

Eating and drinking

Your young child needs a variety of foods to ensure that he or she grows and develops healthily. If you are breastfeeding, feeding on demand will help to fulfil your child's nutritional needs, although you may need to supplement breast milk with bottle feeding at times when your baby's blood glucose is low. If low blood glucose is a constant problem, reducing your child's insulin dose will be helpful.

As you introduce your child to more foods, you will need to include those that contain complex carbohydrate, such as bread, pasta, and potatoes. As your child grows, he or she will need to eat enough carbohydrate at mealtimes and throughout the day to keep his or her blood glucose level in the recommended range (see p.157). Snacks between meals could include fruit juice or milkshakes, cereal bars, crumpets, or fruit.

Your child may be fussy about food at times and his or her eating pattern may vary a lot. This can be frustrating when you want to encourage your child to eat in order to prevent him or her from having a hypo.

If your child refuses food, keep calm. Have an alternative prepared – perhaps a meal or snack that you know your child particularly likes – that will tempt him or her to eat. Be careful not to offer more than one or two choices though: if your child learns that he or she can command many more options, your mealtimes could become a battleground.

You won't do your child any harm if some meals are higher in fat or sugar than others. It is the overall content of his or her food intake that matters. For example, you can compensate for a lunch of fish fingers, chips, and cake by giving your child fruit as a snack later, or a salad or chopped vegetables and a baked potato for tea.

Bedtime snacks

You need to make sure that your child has eaten enough of an evening meal to keep his or her blood glucose from falling overnight, especially if he or she usually sleeps through until morning. If you don't think your child has had enough food and you can't fit in a snack before bedtime, you may need to test your child's blood glucose later in the evening in case he or she becomes hypoglycaemic. If necessary, give your child a drink or easy-to-eat snack. If low blood glucose becomes a regular event, you may need to reduce your child's insulin dose at the evening mealtime. As your child grows older and the time between his or her evening meal and bedtime gets longer, you can start a routine of a snack before he or she goes to bed.

Eating out

There is no reason why you shouldn't eat out as a family when your child has diabetes, whether at a restaurant or a friend's house. Fast food, take-aways, and party food are all good sources of carbohydrate even if they contain too much fat, salt, and sugar, to be good for your child on a regular basis. If you are not sure what food will be on offer or when, pack an emergency supply of foods you know your child will eat (in addition to glucose and longer-acting, carbohydrate-containing food to treat a hypo).

Blood glucose control

Keeping good control of your child's blood glucose level is essential right from the start: what you do now can make a difference to his or her health as an adult and reduce the risk of long-term complications such as eye, kidney, and nerve problems. Good blood glucose control is also important for healthy growth in young children – a high blood glucose level can reduce the effect of growth hormones. Good control for young children is the same as for anyone else with diabetes: the target is for HbA1c levels to be 7 per cent or below (see p.66) and blood glucose test results of 4–7 millimoles per litre most of the time.

You won't always be able to achieve results in this range, but by keeping records of your child's blood glucose test results, you will probably become expert

Practical tips

SUPERVISING YOUR CHILD'S FOOD INTAKE

● Mealtimes are important for social as well as for nutritional reasons – don't make them a carbohydrate battleground! All young children will eat when they are hungry.

● Don't worry if your child doesn't eat healthy food at every meal – it's the overall balance that matters.

● If you're having problems, ask your health professional about ways of matching your child's insulin to his or her current eating pattern.

FAST FOODS
Most children enjoy chips, which, although high in fat, won't do any harm if eaten every so often. If you cook chips at home, you can reduce fat by choosing oven-bake varieties.

Myth OR
TRUTH?

MYTH
You don't have to worry about good diabetes control until your child gets older.

TRUTH
However young your child is when he or she develops diabetes, good control is essential from the start – and is associated with better health in later life. Children are not protected from the effects of poor blood glucose control even though complications might not show until they are adults.

at identifying patterns of highs or lows and working out what to do about them. Taking action as soon as you notice a pattern of blood glucose levels outside the recommended range will limit the effect.

Testing your child's blood glucose level and giving insulin injections may be hard for you, especially at first, but these tasks are essential. To attain the best diabetes control possible, you will need to test your child's blood glucose regularly before and/or after meals and whenever your child engages in a new or unusual activity. You can then adjust your child's treatment, activity, or food intake according to the results.

Identifying patterns
Any changes you make to your child's treatment, activity, or food intake should be based on a pattern of results rather than an individual test result. For example, if your child has a blood glucose reading of more than 10 millimoles per litre at lunchtime for three consecutive days, this is a pattern for which you should try to

find a cause. Ask yourself questions, such as "Is he or she eating or drinking anything different at the moment?", "Has he or she been less active than usual?", or "Is he or she unwell?". Once you identify the cause, you can take action – for the situation described above, you might change what your child is eating for breakfast. If you can't find an obvious reason for high readings, your child may simply need more insulin to match his or her growth – an increase in his or her morning dose is probably necessary for this situation.

Follow up any action with a test to find out whether or not a change has worked. (For more information on making adjustments, see pp.90–95.)

Even if your child has a slightly high blood glucose level and seems well, don't allow this to continue for more than a few days. A higher than normal blood glucose level for longer than this could increase the chance of your child feeling unwell or being at risk of long-term complications when he or she is older.

Good diabetes control also entails avoiding low readings that could lead to hypos (see pp.102–109). Your child is certain to have some hypos, but serious or long-lasting episodes can be frightening for you both. You can prevent these by keeping your child's blood glucose above 4 millimoles per litre.

There will be periods when it is very difficult to keep your child's blood glucose level within the ideal range, particularly as your child

My experience

"Our 8-year-old has had diabetes since he was 4. We have tried most types of insulin – from one injection a day to multiple doses, from half a unit at a time to several units. It's trial and error. You need patience and perseverance." IAIN

COMMENT The insulin requirements of a growing child change constantly. You will need to try different insulins and regimens from time to time to find one that best suits your child at a particular stage of development.

grows older, bigger, and takes part in new activities. Sometimes your child might need a change of insulin type or regimen (see pp.87–95). Discuss the options with your health professional. You can also be certain that you'll need to make changes again before too long!

Tests and injections

Although you might find it difficult to inject your child every day, he or she needs insulin to live, and blood glucose tests will always be part of his or her everyday life. The exact times you test and give insulin each day will vary but will follow a general pattern. For example, your child will need an insulin injection around one or more of his or her mealtimes and blood glucose tests either just before or two hours after meals.

The doses of insulin you give will also vary. For up to two years after diagnosis, your child may experience a "honeymoon period", which means that he or she is likely to need only very small doses of insulin. Once this period is over, your child will need more insulin. You may also need to increase the insulin dose often when your child has a growth spurt. Learning to adjust your child's insulin is part of learning to live with diabetes, and your health professional will help you with this.

Coping with tantrums

There will be times when your child is not willing to have an injection or to have his or her blood glucose tested. Think about how you encourage your child to take care of other aspects of his or her health, such as bathing or toothbrushing, and try to incorporate diabetes care into his or her routine in the same way. Bear in mind that very young children may fiercely resist having an injection or test, but are easily distracted immediately afterwards.

Even if you sometimes feel guilty about giving your child an injection or doing a blood test when he or she is upset, be careful about the kind of reward you give afterwards. Having a cuddle, reading a book, or playing with a favourite toy together can help your child to link injection or test time with a pleasurable experience, but rewards such as new activities, new toys, or even food can be difficult to deliver every day.

Doing a blood test on yourself or inserting one of your child's clean needles into your skin when you are alone may help you to understand what testing and injecting feels like in reality.

Dealing with hypos

Hypos are a side effect of insulin treatment so your child will have them from time to time, especially if you are keeping good control of his or her diabetes. If your child is too young to talk, the symptoms of hypoglycaemia will be difficult to recognize at first and you will need to be alert for signs that come on quickly, such as becoming very uncoordinated, sweaty, pale, silent, or staring into space. Your

Practical tips

TESTING OR INJECTING A RELUCTANT CHILD

- Explain what you are going to do and do it immediately. Don't say that you'll do something "in 5 minutes" – this will increase any sense of anxiety.
- Hold your child firmly and securely on your knee as you test or inject.
- Ask other family members to help if necessary.
- Allow your child to help if he or she wants to (and is old enough).
- Cuddle and praise your child when the test or injection is finished.
- Afterwards, quickly get back to what the two of you were doing beforehand.

TREATING A SEVERE HYPO

If severe hypoglycaemia is untreated, there is a risk that your child could become unconscious or have a fit. A fit doesn't mean that your child has epilepsy; it is the brain's reaction to insufficient glucose. You will need to keep calm and take the following measures to help your child recover.

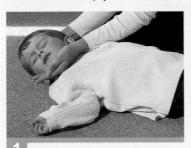

1 If your child is having a fit, make sure his mouth is clear to breathe. If you are still worried, call an ambulance.

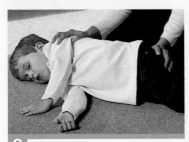

2 If your child can breathe normally, lie him on his side or hold him with his head tilted back slightly to keep his airway clear.

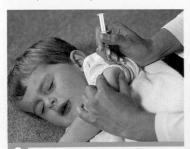

3 Prepare, or ask someone else to prepare, a glucagon injection (see p.109) and give it to your child in his arm, buttock, or leg. Don't try to give him anything to eat or drink.

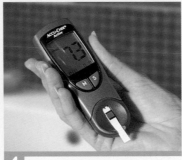

4 When your child has regained consciousness, he might vomit as a result of the glucagon injection. Sit him up and check his blood glucose level as soon as it is practical to do so.

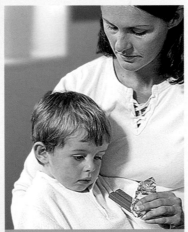

5 Once he is more alert, give him some food or drink that contains carbohydrate to keep his blood glucose level raised.

6 Check his blood glucose level every half hour until it is above 4 millimoles per litre and stay with him until you are both feeling better.

child's warning signs are individual but tend to be the same each time, so it's important to learn what they are. You also need to be aware that your child could have a severe hypo if he or she:

- Has been very physically active but hasn't had less insulin or more food to compensate.
- Eats less than usual over several meals.
- Has had too much insulin.
- Becomes overheated, for example, in hot weather.
- Has a vomiting illness.

A blood glucose test will confirm whether your child's blood glucose level has fallen below 4 millimoles per litre, which means that he or she is hypoglycaemic.

If you can't do a test, and you think your child is hypoglycaemic because of his or her symptoms, it won't do any harm to give your baby a breastfeed or bottle feed, or your young child glucose tablets, a glucose drink, or glucose gel (see p.106) to raise his or her blood glucose level. The sooner you treat a hypo, the sooner your child will recover.

Because hypos can be unpredictable, it's useful to keep glucose tablets or a sugary drink to hand to treat them. You can also limit the risk of hypos by giving your child a carbohydrate snack at bedtime or waking him or her for a feed or snack during the night. During the day, regular feeds or meals and snacks will help to balance insulin doses. If your child eats much less than usual at a mealtime or over several mealtimes, you may need to reduce his or her next dose of insulin.

If you know that your child will be particularly active, such as at a party, or running around outside, you can give him or her more to eat or a reduced insulin dose beforehand. Extra activity at any time can cause your child's blood glucose level to fall several hours later. To avoid serious hypos as a result, particularly at night, give your child extra food over a few hours following his or her activity.

Coping with illness

From time to time, your child, like any other, will become unwell. Children are not more likely to be ill just because they have diabetes, but if their diabetes is not well controlled and they have a high blood glucose level over a period of time, they may be more prone to infections. This is because glucose-rich blood provides an ideal environment for germs to multiply.

When your child has diabetes, any illness can affect his or her blood glucose level and vice versa. Unlike adults, whose blood glucose always rises during illness, children's blood glucose can either rise or fall, so their doses of insulin may need to be increased or decreased. The golden rule is to continue giving your child his or her insulin every day and not to stop for any reason. This is to prevent diabetic ketoacidosis (see p.113). Even if your child is not

eating, he or she must continue to have insulin, although you may need to give very small doses. Doing more blood glucose tests when your child is unwell will help you decide how much insulin to give. Discussing how to deal with illness with your health professional and having information to hand about what to do will help you cope when your child becomes unwell.

To care for your sick child, give sugar-free drinks to keep him or her hydrated and test his or her blood glucose level at least four times a day. If your child has a high temperature, remove most of his or her clothing, and use a facecloth moistened with tepid water to cool his or her skin. Your child should also have plenty of cool drinks and may need a temperature-lowering medicine from your health professional or pharmacy.

Young children can become unwell quickly, which can make their blood glucose level difficult to control. If you can't bring your child's blood glucose under control while he or she is ill, contact your health professional for advice.

If your child is vomiting and cannot keep any food or drink down at all, take him or her to a hospital casualty department immediately or call an ambulance. In this situation, your child will need insulin and fluid via an infusion to prevent him or her from becoming seriously ill with diabetic ketoacidosis (see p.113).

If your child is vomiting and cannot keep any food or drink down at all, take him or her to a hospital casualty department immediately or call an ambulance.

School-age children

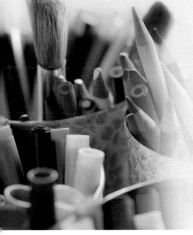

Whether your child has recently been diagnosed with diabetes or has had diabetes from a young age, his or her school years present new challenges. As your child grows and becomes more independent, it is important to encourage his or her involvement in diabetes care, with initial supervision of injections and testing. You also need to develop a system of diabetes care that fits in with a school routine; obtaining the support of school staff will help to keep your child's diabetes well controlled.

Diabetes, your child, and you

Children between the ages of five and 12 who develop diabetes are most likely to have Type 1 diabetes. Although cases of Type 2 diabetes in school-age children have been found, they are extremely rare. The symptoms of diabetes, including passing a lot of urine, thirst, and weight loss are the same in school-age children as in adults (see pp.18–19). You might notice that your child starts to wet the bed, is always drinking, and is much more tired than usual.

A school-age child with diabetes needs insulin injections, blood tests, and a balanced food intake that includes plenty of carbohydrate foods. A child with diabetes can do everything that any other child can do, but good blood glucose control is important to keep him or her healthy

A child with diabetes can do everything any other child can do, but blood glucose control is important to keep him or her healthy.

now and to prevent complications associated with diabetes in the future. Good blood glucose control is also important to ensure your child's healthy physical development, because a consistently high blood glucose level can reduce the effectiveness of growth hormone.

As soon as your child starts to go to school, he or she will be more independent, will be asking lots of questions, and making new friends. Your child is also likely to be very active, for example, going out more to other people's houses, and enjoying school trips and parties. As a parent, it's important to balance caring for your child's diabetes with allowing him or her to simply get on and grow up. You can also help your child on the path to self-sufficiency by encouraging his or her involvement in diabetes care. Until your child is older, you will be the best judge of what he or she is

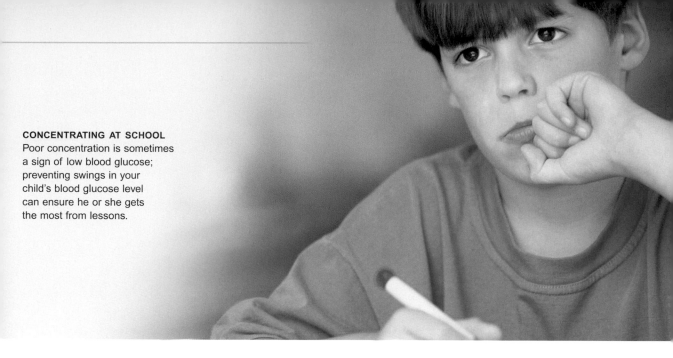

CONCENTRATING AT SCHOOL
Poor concentration is sometimes a sign of low blood glucose; preventing swings in your child's blood glucose level can ensure he or she gets the most from lessons.

capable of and when. Sometimes your child will want to be involved in his or her diabetes care and sometimes he or she won't. This is normal, and adapting to it is part of being a parent.

If your child has recently been diagnosed with diabetes, you will have many different feelings, worries, and questions. You may feel shocked at first, and possibly overwhelmed. You will have the opportunity of discussing the way you feel with a health professional. You may also find it very helpful to get together and share experiences, successes, and worries with other parents of children with diabetes.

Telling other people

How many people you tell and how much information you provide about your child's diabetes is a personal decision and depends to a large extent on how involved other people are in caring for your child's diabetes.

■ **TALKING TO TEACHERS** Your child's teachers may know little about diabetes, so you may wish to arrange a meeting with them to explain your child's needs. Your health professional can accompany you to advise school staff about diabetes and address their concerns. The more information and clear

Q My daughter has had diabetes for six months and has gradually needed less and less insulin. Will she stop needing it altogether?

A It sounds as though your daughter is experiencing what is called the "honeymoon period", which can last anything up to 2 years after Type 1 diabetes is diagnosed. During this time, the pancreas seems to recover a little and starts producing insulin again, so only small doses of injected insulin are needed. However, at some stage within 2 years, your daughter's insulin-producing cells will stop working altogether and she will require larger doses of insulin again.

MANAGING YOUR CHILD'S INSULIN

• Make sure that your child hasn't had so many snacks or drinks that he or she can't eat at mealtimes. If you're worried about hypos between meals or at school, you may need to reduce your child's insulin doses rather than overdo the snacks.

• If you can't predict how much or when your child will eat, you may wish to use an insulin that you can give up to 15 minutes after a meal. Ask your health professional for advice.

• It's the overall control of your child's diabetes that matters, not a single blood glucose result. These won't be perfect all the time – no one's are!

instructions you can provide, the more confident teachers and staff are likely to feel about their ability to care for your child at school.

One way to communicate with teachers about your child's diabetes is to use a notebook. You and your child's teacher can write in the book to keep in touch and share relevant information. For example, you might want to tell the teacher that your child's blood glucose level is high that day; or the teacher might notice that your child needs to go to the toilet more often.

Your child may have a hypo at school if he or she is not able to have a meal or snack at the usual time, has not had enough to eat, or has used up more energy than normal, such as during an extra sports lesson or a particularly energetic game at break time. You will need to warn staff that a hypo might occur immediately or an hour or two later, and that your child will need to take or be given glucose – in the form of tablets or a drink – quickly. Your child should keep emergency supplies to treat a hypo with him or her at all times. You should also tell school staff what to do should your child become unconscious as a result of hypoglycaemia (see pp.102–109).

Naturally you will want to prevent your child from experiencing hypos at school. However, keeping his or her blood glucose level above the recommended 4–7 millimoles per litre in order to prevent a hypo will

not benefit your child in the long term because it may make him or her more prone to illness and it increases the risk of long-term complications. If you are worried about hypos at school, or they are happening often, your child may need a different insulin regimen. Talk to your health professional about the choices available.

Eating and drinking

The principles of healthy eating (see pp.30–43) are the same for a child with diabetes as for any other child – meals should be based on complex carbohydrates with some protein, and fat, sugar, and salt in moderation. Also, encourage your child to eat several portions of fruit and vegetables a day.

In general, your child needs three meals a day, plus a morning, afternoon, and bedtime snack. Snacks between meals will top up your child's energy and balance with his or her insulin to prevent hypos. However, because your child's appetite will vary, you'll have to be flexible about how much he or she eats.

On some days, for example, you may need to give your child an extra snack to compensate for an unusually small lunch. On other days, he or she might be particularly hungry at dinner time and ask for extra helpings. Learning to adjust your child's insulin dose to accommodate new eating patterns can be very helpful.

If your child is going to be particularly active, on school sports day, for example, he or she will need an extra glucose snack beforehand and may need extra food several hours later (see p.169).

Eating at school

There is no reason why your child shouldn't have school meals. School menus are usually based on healthy eating guidelines, so your child should be offered a variety of good foods.

If your child is not willing or able to eat enough carbohydrate at lunchtime, you may need to ask teachers and catering staff if it is possible to offer alternative foods. You should also discuss whether your child may need to be among the first to be served at lunchtime, or be in the same sitting every day, in order to prevent a hypo.

Your child will need a snack mid-morning and at afternoon break to balance his or her morning insulin. There may be times when your child needs to eat a snack earlier, such as if he or she feels hypo, or break time is delayed. Make sure school staff are aware of this and will allow your child to quietly get on with eating when necessary. Small, easy-to-eat snacks are especially useful at these times.

You might prefer to give your child packed lunches, so that you can choose healthy foods that he or she likes. Your child can also play a part in choosing and making packed lunches. You could include any of the following foods in a packed lunch or as snacks.

- Bread, such as bagels or finger rolls with low-fat fillings, rice cakes, teacakes, crumpets, or breadsticks.
- Low-fat crisps or small cheese biscuits.
- Fruit – dried, tinned in natural juice, or fresh – in small easy-to-eat pieces, if necessary.
- Individual packs of cereal with semi-skimmed milk.
- Cereal bars.
- Fruit yoghurt.
- Milkshake made with semi-skimmed milk and fresh fruit or fruit yoghurt.
- Two or three plain biscuits, such as ginger biscuits, or crackers.

Whether your child has school meals or packed lunches, knowing the answers to the following questions will help you to plan his or her food intake throughout the school day:
- What time does the school day start and finish?
- Are children allowed to eat at morning and afternoon break times, and how often are breaks delayed?

You might prefer to give your child packed lunches, so that you can choose healthy foods that he or she likes.

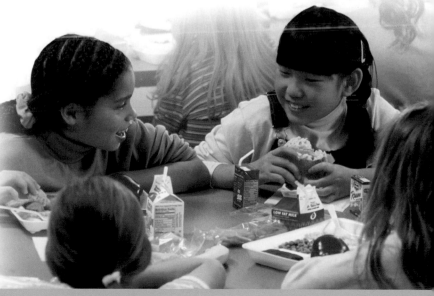

EATING AT LUNCHTIME
It's important to make sure that your child eats enough carbohydrate-containing foods at lunchtime to prevent hypos later in the day.

Alert your child's teacher to the possibility of a hypo occurring on a school trip, and check that your child will be allowed to eat if necessary.

PARTY FOOD
No child wants to miss out on treats such as birthday cake, and although an occasional sweet feast may increase your child's blood glucose level temporarily, it won't do any harm.

● What time is lunch; is it different for children who have school meals and those who have packed lunches?
● When does your child have a sports lesson, and how often do unplanned physical activities take place?

Eating at friends' houses

Your child may be invited to other children's houses for meals or parties. Because these are not everyday events, your child can enjoy high-fat or sugary snacks and cakes, even if this causes his or her blood glucose level to rise temporarily. If you are concerned that your child's blood glucose will rise too much, however, you could ask the person in charge to have sugar-free drinks available or provide them yourself.

If your child tends to rush around with friends playing party games, for example, the energy he or she uses will balance out any extra food he or she has eaten. If your child is quieter and less active, he or she may need a little extra insulin that day. However, a single occasion with high blood glucose will not cause damage in the long term. It is a raised blood glucose level for more than a week or two that can be harmful.

School trips

On school trips, when meals might be earlier or later than usual, your child will need a few extra snacks and hypo supplies in case of delays. It's worth reminding your child not to eat all his or her snacks at once and not to share them with friends. On these occasions, it will not do your child any harm to eat more than usual even if it causes his or her blood glucose to rise for that day.

Alert your child's teacher to the possibility of a hypo occurring on a school trip, and check that your child will be allowed to eat if necessary. Remind the person in charge that your child's blood glucose level might rise as a result of excitement and so he or she may need to go to the toilet more often or be extra thirsty (see

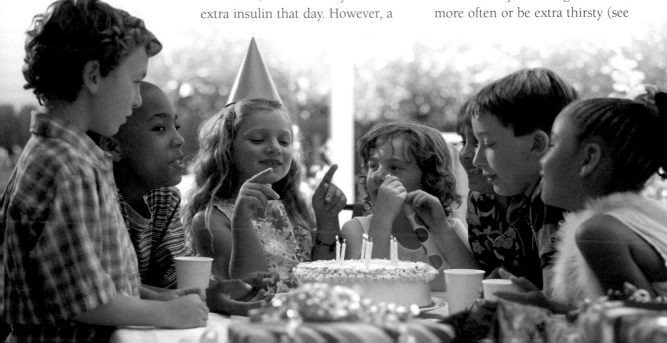

Hyperglycaemia, pp.110–113). Before the school trip, make sure that you have the following information.

- Leaving and returning times and whether these are likely to be delayed.
- Arrangements for snacks and meals.
- Name of the person in charge – is it the usual teacher or someone else?
- Arrangements for contacting parents if there should be a problem.

Blood glucose control

Good control of your child's diabetes means that he or she should have blood glucose readings of 4–7 millimoles per litre most of the time and an HbA1c level (see p.66) of around 7 per cent. The more often you can achieve these levels, the greater the chances of preventing long-term complications when your child grows up. Maintaining these levels means testing your child's blood glucose level regularly and adjusting his or her treatment, activity, or food intake according to the results. Identifying and treating patterns is more useful than acting on an individual result (see pp.62–75).

Changing routines, activity levels, and growing rates all affect blood glucose and insulin needs, so your child's blood glucose readings won't always be within the ideal range. A week or two outside this range from time to time won't do any harm, but a consistently high blood glucose level increases your child's risk of health problems later in life. A slightly higher blood glucose level won't necessarily

make your child feel any different. He or she will only have symptoms, such as thirst or tiredness, with a glucose level of 10 millimoles per litre or more. In fact, your child's body can adjust to a slightly higher glucose level so that he or she may feel hypo even if his or her blood glucose is within the recommended range.

Unfortunately, children are less enthusiastic about aiming for normal readings if this makes them feel hypo. The way to combat this is to keep testing and adjusting insulin or food to achieve a normal blood glucose level for long enough – a few days at least – for your child to feel well at these levels (see pp.90–95 for more information on adjusting doses).

Tests and injections

Your child needs tests and injections every day to keep his or her diabetes under good control. To help your child learn that caring for his or her diabetes is an important part of the daily routine, it's a good idea to treat tests and injections like any other health-related activity, such as hand washing, hair- or toothbrushing.

Practical tips

INVOLVING CHILDREN IN DIABETES CARE

- Explain simply and clearly to your child what insulin is for and why he or she needs to learn how to test and inject, so that it becomes a familiar story.
- If your child stops doing his or her own tests or injections, take over for a few days. Children like to be independent, so will take charge again eventually!
- To maintain or refresh your child's interest in his or her diabetes, consider a change of insulin device or blood glucose meter from time to time – there are types available to suit all tastes.
- Make sure that your child carries a supply of glucose and some form of identification at all times.

My experience

"I took care of my diabetes from the age of 11. I tried many insulins to see what suited me best and lots of blood glucose meters to find which gave me the results quickest." SHELLEY

COMMENT Some children are able to manage their own diabetes from an early age and make decisions about what's important to them, such as how to make it easier to do tests or injections. There is a wide range of equipment that is easy to use and appealing to children.

PREVENTING PROBLEMS

• Keep a record of all your child's daily blood glucose results, so you can identify patterns and decide if anything needs to change.

• Injecting constantly in the same site causes lumps and also means insulin isn't absorbed properly. Change your child's injection site regularly and teach him or her to do this him- or herself.

INJECTION TIMES
Sometimes children are happy to take responsibility for their own injections; at other times they may lose all interest in looking after their diabetes and you will need to take charge for a little while.

There is no ideal age for your child to start doing his or her own blood tests and injections. He or she may want to start doing it at primary school or may not show an interest until secondary school. Your child might be keener to do one or the other first, or need your help at some times more than others. You can help most by going along with what your child feels able to do, and making sure that tests and injections are performed with as little fuss as possible, whoever does them.

Involving children as much as possible in working out what their test results mean and what changes you need to make to their insulin dose, food intake, or activity levels will help them towards taking responsibility for their own diabetes. It is important to praise your child for looking after his or her diabetes well, but avoid allowing him or her to negotiate testing or injection times too much as this can easily create a frustrating daily battle.

Occasionally, you or your child will need to change the type or timing of his or her insulin and the frequency of tests, perhaps because your child is having a growth spurt, eating more or less of certain foods, has a different routine at school, or has started to socialize more outside your home. Ask your health professional to help you choose the best system from the wide range of insulins, injection devices, and blood glucose meters available.

Dealing with hypos

Trying to keep good control of your child's diabetes will inevitably mean that, from time to time, he or she will become hypoglycaemic (when blood glucose falls below 4 millimoles per litre). The signs that your child is hypo will be similar each time, so it is important that you, your child, and teachers learn to recognize them.

The older your child, the more able he or she will be to take action or tell someone when symptoms occur. Your child should carry glucose at all times and, if he or she is able to recognize the warning signs of a hypo, should learn to take glucose before a hypo becomes severe. Sometimes, however, your child will be unaware of the signs or won't tell you how he or she feels, so you and

Q What will happen if my daughter has a hypo in the night that I don't know about?

A Your daughter will wake up naturally in the morning. This is because her insulin will wear off overnight and her liver will also react to the hypo, by converting stored glycogen into glucose and releasing it into her bloodstream. As a result, your daughter's blood glucose level could be very high in the morning, and she may also have a headache and feel tired. You can prevent hypos at night by giving your child extra food or less insulin in the evening.

your child's teachers need to be alert for sudden changes in behaviour, such as your child being particularly naughty, argumentative, aggressive, or very sleepy. A blood test will confirm hypoglycaemia but if you can't test, you won't do any harm by treating what seems to be a hypo straight away (see pp.106–108).

Hypos can also occur some time after your child has been physically active because his or her injected insulin will continue to work after the glucose in his or her body has been used for energy. However, it is important that your child is active because exercise helps to keep his or her heart healthy, maintains a healthy body weight, and keeps blood pressure and blood fat levels in the recommended range. So if you are worried about hypos, try changing the time of your child's insulin injection or reducing the dose before activity. If the activity is unplanned, give your child an extra carbohydrate snack. If the activity lasts longer than an hour, your child may need extra glucose in the form of a drink or tablet during the activity, too.

Although you will want to protect your child against hypos, avoid the temptation to keep blood glucose consistently too high (above 10 millimoles per litre) in an effort to prevent them. There is no guarantee that such measures will work because insulin levels in the bloodstream and the amount of energy used up by your child throughout the day may vary a lot. In addition, a high blood

> **My experience**
>
> *"It has been helpful to have a very good multi-disciplinary paediatric diabetes team at the end of a phone for help and advice. The team knows us as a family and that's great."* IAIN
>
> **COMMENT** Caring for a child with diabetes can sometimes be a challenge for the whole family, so it is reassuring to be able to contact health professionals who know you and your child and understand your situation.

glucose level can produce symptoms as well as put your child at risk of health complications in the future.

Life at school

Your child's diabetes will not affect his or her ability to learn or to take part in school activities. Provided he or she is allowed to eat meals and snacks when necessary and you can plan for food needs, testing, and injections, school life shouldn't present any obstacles.

Depending on your child's age, he or she may be able to do blood tests during the school day. If your child has an insulin injection at lunchtime, you may need go to school to supervise or give the injection. If this proves difficult, ask your health professional to help you devise an insulin and testing system that can be used outside school hours.

If school staff are worried about your child's diabetes, they may be unwilling to allow him or her to participate in some activities. If you believe that this is the case, talk to the headteacher and ask for your health professional's help to work out a solution.

Your child should carry glucose at all times and, if he or she is able to recognize the warning signs of a hypo, should learn to take glucose before a hypo becomes severe.

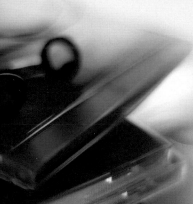

Teenagers and young adults

This is the time that most childhood diabetes begins. Adolescence is a time of change; a teenager with diabetes not only has peer pressures, exams, and the effects of hormones to contend with – but also blood glucose control. As a parent, you need to be supportive. As a teenager, you need to cope with your feelings, eat and drink healthily when you can, and look after your diabetes in ways that suit your lifestyle. You also need to know how smoking, alcohol, and drugs can affect your diabetes.

Diabetes, your teenager, and you

Teenagers and young adults who develop diabetes are likely to have Type 1 diabetes, previously known as juvenile onset diabetes. However, Type 2 diabetes, which usually affects older people, is now being found in children and teenagers, too. Although only a few teenagers have been diagnosed with Type 2 diabetes in the UK, in the US, the numbers are greater, and

rising rapidly. The rise in Type 2 diabetes among the young is believed to be linked to sedentary lifestyles and increasing levels of obesity. As many as 80 per cent of young people with Type 2 diabetes may be overweight at the time of diagnosis. If your teenager has developed Type 2 diabetes or MODY (a form of diabetes similar to Type 2; see p.16), this needs to be managed in the same way as Type 2 diabetes in an older person.

The symptoms of Type 1 diabetes, including passing a lot of urine, thirst, and weight loss, are the same in teenagers as in adults (see pp.18–19). Symptoms can come on very quickly – over a few days or a week – and you might notice that your teenager is more tired than usual and getting up in the night to go to the toilet or have a drink.

A teenager with Type 1 diabetes needs insulin injections, blood tests, and a balanced food intake that

---

My experience

"I thought I must have done something wrong. I felt upset and confused ... I was worried about my mum as she was frightened, too. Then I met other people who were going through the same thing and I didn't feel quite so alone." JANE

COMMENT The feelings you have when you are first diagnosed with diabetes as a teenager can be very negative. It's reassuring to know that you aren't the only one and to talk to teenagers in the same position.

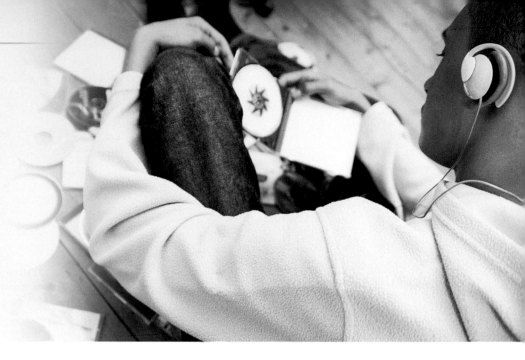

DEALING WITH DIABETES
It can be difficult to deal with your diabetes when you are a teenager or young adult. Taking time out to come to terms with your feelings and developing a strategy for fitting diabetes care into your busy life can help you feel more positive.

includes plenty of carbohydrate foods. Type 2 diabetes or MODY may be treated with healthy eating and physical activity, followed by tablets and insulin injections when necessary. Whatever type of diabetes your teenager has, good diabetes care now is important to keep your teenager in the best of health and to prevent complications associated with diabetes in the future.

Whether your teenager has recently been diagnosed with diabetes or has had diabetes from a very young age, teenage years bring both challenges and pressures. The transition into adulthood is a time of physical and emotional change and growth, and the effects of hormones can be great. Relationships with peers can also be difficult at this time and the added pressure of exams or working life may not help. Having diabetes can complicate your teenager's life even further and cause you worry as a

parent, but there are ways of working together to make the process of growing up as trouble-free as possible.

Out of concern and love, you may be tempted to try to keep control of your teenager's diabetes, but this is virtually impossible. It is your teenager's diabetes, and he or she must eventually take full responsibility for it. Try to develop a supportive rather than a controlling role.

Teenagers still need, and will respond to, rules and boundaries, even though they might argue about them endlessly. Be firm and consistent and treat diabetes care as you would any other aspect of your teenager's life that requires rules, such as coming home at a certain time or keeping his or her bedroom tidy. For example, you might insist that your teenager performs a minimum number of blood tests per day or per week; that he or she does not go out until he or she has taken

> Good diabetes care now is important to keep your teenager in the best of health and to prevent complications associated with diabetes in the future.

their insulin and eaten; that he or she eats high-fat or high-sugar foods only two or three times a week; or that he or she attends clinic visits without argument. The more you involve teenagers in making decisions about what they are going to do, the more likely it is that they will stick to what has been agreed.

No parent is perfect and your relationship with your teenager and his or her diabetes will not always go smoothly. However, a teenager who is doing most or even some things that are important in looking after his or her diabetes deserves praise and encouragement. If you are worried that your teenager is not doing enough and none of your ideas seem to work, you will need help from family, friends, or your health professional. When your teenager doesn't seem to listen to you, he or she will often be more receptive to friends, so ask for the support of anyone you think will encourage your teenager to keep on top of his or her diabetes management. You can also contact health professionals who work with teenagers.

As a parent, you want your child to grow up healthy and happy, and able to make his or her way in the world. On the other hand, your child probably wants to live for the moment and be one of the crowd. He or she may rebel against authority, experiment with activities, and test out different relationships. How teenagers treat their diabetes varies,

TALKING TO TEENAGERS
Good communication involves listening as well as talking, so it's important to give your teenager a fair hearing, even if you don't necessarily agree with what's being said.

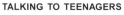

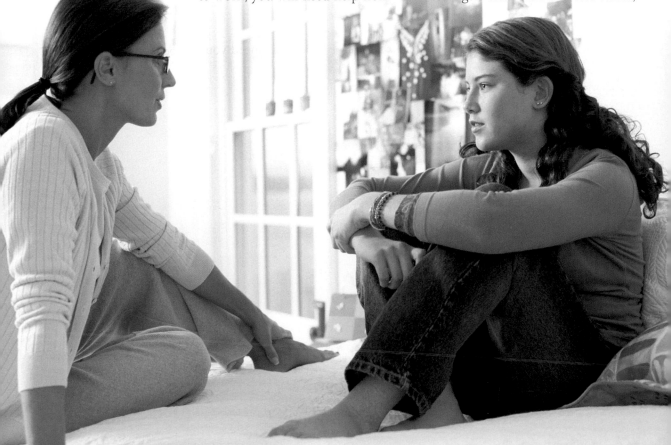

but it is likely to be similar to the way in which they treat other aspects of their lives. So they may realize the importance of the day-to-day tasks of caring for their diabetes, and fit them in without huge effort. On the other hand, they may see diabetes as setting them apart from their friends and so try to make it less obvious by ignoring it or doing little in the way of testing or eating healthily.

At the same time, your teenager's diabetes will be changing. The effect of hormones is likely to increase the amount of insulin he or she needs throughout adolescence. In addition, the pressures of taking exams or starting work, developing sexually, and possibly experimenting with alcohol or drugs will all affect his or her blood glucose level. So home blood tests and contact with your health professional continue to be important.

Talking to your teenager

Communication with your teenager may be straightforward and open or may sometimes consist of one-word answers, arguments, or even shouting matches or battles of will. In general, any talking is good, but the calmer, the better. Even if your teenager seems to reject your every word, the lines of communication must remain open for when he or she is ready to talk. There is no reason why you shouldn't let your teenager know what you think and feel about his or her diabetes, although it may help to choose a time when you feel your child is at his or her most receptive.

Your feelings as a teenager

When you have diabetes it seems as though there is a lot to do to look after yourself. It can seem to get in the way of your day-to-day life and you won't always want to do your blood tests and injections, or think about when and what you're going to eat. The good news is that you are normal – no one, whether they have diabetes or not, can always do everything they are meant to in relation to their health.

The not-so-good news is that if you regularly don't take care of your diabetes you are very likely to be storing up problems for later on. You probably think that developing problems in 20 years' time sounds a long way off, but even then you will still be under 40 and you'll need your eyesight, healthy feet and kidneys, and a strong heart for the rest of your life. You don't have to be perfect all the time to make sure this is the case for you, but you do need to work at it some of the time.

If you've just been diagnosed

You should be feeling a lot better now that you are taking insulin, and learning a lot of new information. Your health professional will be in touch with you regularly and you probably feel quite keen to do all your tests and injections and eat the right things. Your friends and family will be paying you a lot of attention at the moment, partly out of worry about you and partly because it's all new to them, too. You will find that, as you get used to having diabetes, the novelty will wear off and you might become a bit bored or fed up with testing and injections, especially if you are feeling well again. However, it's important to try to find ways to keep going with your diabetes care.

If you've had diabetes for a while

Diabetes sometimes gets in the way of what you want to do and means that you can't behave as spontaneously as your friends. It can be very tempting to ignore your diabetes when you feel like this, and to let your blood glucose run at a level that stops you feeling hypo but also isn't high enough to give you symptoms of high blood glucose, such as passing urine frequently, thirst, and tiredness.

This can help you to fit in with your friends, but it can make you more prone to infections in the short

> **You might become a bit bored or fed up with testing and injections ... so it's important to find ways to keep going with your diabetes care.**

Q **Can having diabetes stunt your growth?**

A Provided your diabetes is well controlled, it should not affect your growth. However, if your blood glucose level is consistently high, you may not reach your full height because your growth hormone will not work effectively if there isn't enough insulin in your bloodstream. This is one reason why you need to keep your blood glucose level within the recommended range as much as possible.

term and do some damage to your blood vessels in the long run.

There are lots of different insulins, devices, and testing kits available that can make life easier for you. Your health professional is there to help you work out the most effective system of treatment. You may need to try out different insulin regimens to find one that suits you (see pp.87–90).

Dealing with strong feelings

You might find that you have very strong feelings about having diabetes – anger, resentment, or hate, for example. You might also feel upset or guilty. These emotions are normal, especially if you have recently found out you have diabetes. But if you think that your feelings are disrupting your studies, work, or family life, you may need to share them with someone else.

Your health professional will probably ask you how you're feeling when you visit and will listen and discuss your feelings with you, or you might prefer to talk to someone else. A school counsellor, youth club leader, a friend, or a friend's parent might be easier to talk to honestly and openly about your diabetes.

Having diabetes can affect the way you see yourself, too. Because insulin builds up the tissues in your body, it can make you put on weight. There are ways to limit this, for example by eating healthily and being physically active, but you might worry about it a lot. You may think that if you don't take your insulin, you won't put on weight – you may even lose weight as you might have done before your diabetes was controlled. But this is not a good way to lose weight, and your blood glucose level would soon become so high that you might be at risk of diabetic ketoacidosis (see p.113).

When you feel well, you may also wonder if you really do have diabetes and, as a result, you might decide not to take your insulin or to take only part of your dose (doing this will remind you what happens to your blood glucose level without enough insulin). Also, from time to time, you will simply forget your injection because you are busy with something else.

However, there is a huge difference between missing the occasional dose and regularly having insufficient insulin. If you keep missing injections, your raised blood glucose level will be high enough to make you feel unwell, cause a serious infection, or result in diabetic ketoacidosis, as well as increase your chances of long-term complications.

Managing stress

Getting things into perspective is important – diabetes is for life, but it's not the only thing in your life. Remind yourself that you are doing the best that you can and a short period in which you take less notice of your diabetes won't do you any harm.

My experience

"I had acute depression…stopped caring about life. The doctor put it down to the enormous psychological effect of having diabetes, which I had coped with far too well as a teenager." LOUISE

COMMENT It is very unusual for a teenager to have such serious depression, but sometimes it is healthier to react emotionally to having diabetes than not to react at all. Louise recovered fully and now believes that she might have felt better had she rebelled a little at the time rather than passively accepting her diabetes.

Stress management can be useful – deep breathing, stretching, a walk in the fresh air, or listening to your favourite music can all help you to feel less pressured.

Talking to your family or close friends about all the things you need to do to look after your diabetes can help you feel as though you are sharing the burden, and perhaps help you to think of new ways of fitting your diabetes care into your lifestyle. A local support group for young people with diabetes, where you can share experiences, moans, and laughs, might also help you to feel less isolated.

If you are feeling anxious or depressed, ask your health professional for advice – you might need help to make you feel better about your diabetes and more positive about looking after it. National diabetes organizations, including Diabetes UK, also provide anonymous helplines staffed by people who understand the demands of living with diabetes (see p.218).

● Dancing and having sex
are both forms of physical
activity – so you may need
to adopt strategies to
prevent hypos!

● Don't drive for more than
2 hours without checking
your blood glucose level.
Not only is it dangerous to
have a hypo at the wheel,
but you could also end up
with a restricted licence
or have to stop driving
altogether for a while.

● If you have problem skin,
you can still take antibiotics
and other medicines to
help treat it.

Eating and drinking

Food and drink play an essential part
in keeping your blood glucose under
control, preventing hypos, and
helping you to grow and develop.
Of course, eating and drinking are
part of your social life, too. The more
you can learn about what constitutes
healthy eating and how different foods
affect your blood glucose level, the
better you can adjust your insulin to
suit the food you are eating. No foods
are banned when you have diabetes
and you don't have to eat special
foods, but trying to avoid too many
unhealthy foods and making healthy
choices overall will help you control
your diabetes.

You need to eat carbohydrate-
containing foods regularly to prevent
hypoglycaemia. If your eating pattern
is irregular or the amount you eat
varies a lot, you might need a flexible
insulin regimen so that you can easily
adjust your insulin doses. You can
discuss this with your health
professional who will help you to
work out the best regimen for you.

You may find that some foods make
it difficult to control your blood
glucose no matter what you do
with your insulin. Trying different
insulins and testing equipment, and
experimenting with food and insulin
doses will allow you to adapt to
different situations (see pp.90–95).

Eating healthily is as important for
you as it is for your friends who don't
have diabetes, but just as they do,
you can still have your favourite fast
food, curry, pizza, Chinese, or
puddings and sweets. Sometimes you
may eat a lot of these foods, such as
on holiday, but having them every
day means you will be eating a lot
of extra calories and fat. Basing your
eating on a variety of other foods
such as bread, cereals, fish, and fruit
and vegetables will mean that your
everyday food is low in fat – and this
will protect your heart for the future.
You can find out more about different
meals and how to eat healthily on
pp.30–43.

Blood glucose control

To have good control of your diabetes,
your blood glucose test results need
to be in the range of 4–7 millimoles
per litre most of the time, which
will mean that your HbA1c level
(see p.66) will be around 7 per
cent. You'll have your HbA1c level
tested when you visit your diabetes
health professional – it's an important
test, so this is a good reason to keep
your appointments.

You are unlikely to get all your
blood glucose tests in the ideal range,
partly because this would mean you
have lots of hypos and partly because
taking insulin by injection won't
always keep your blood glucose
balanced as effectively as natural
insulin does. As a result, some of
your test results are likely to be
outside the desired range.

To keep your blood glucose level
as close to the recommended range
as possible, you need to look for
patterns of high or low readings and

work out why they are happening, so that you can make changes to your food, activity, and insulin doses to get your results back on track. You'll need to do this often during your teenage years because hormones such as adrenaline, cortisol, growth hormone, oestrogen, and testosterone, which you produce as you grow and develop, can make your insulin less effective. You will find that you need more insulin at some times than at others. Also, if you're female, you may find that your periods affect your blood glucose level (see p.136).

If you have a consistently high blood glucose level, you'll feel thirsty, tired, and have to pass urine a lot. If you try to keep these symptoms at bay by taking enough insulin, you will be doing a lot towards keeping yourself well for the future.

Your diabetes won't make you less likely to get spots, acne, or greasy skin, but a high blood glucose level can make you more susceptible to infections, including skin infections. So if you do get acne or spots, keeping your blood glucose level well controlled will help prevent them from getting worse.

Tests and injections

Whatever type of insulin you take, you won't always stay on the same dose because life doesn't always stay the same every day. If you didn't have diabetes, your body wouldn't naturally produce the same amount of insulin each day

My experience

"In the past, I haven't always been up to doing lots of monitoring and caring for my diabetes, but at least by going to clinics regularly the professionals were getting some idea about my control, by doing HbA1c readings and checking my feet, kidneys, heart, and eyes." SHELLEY

COMMENT The reality of diabetes is that you don't always feel that you can keep up with its demands. This is why keeping regular appointments with your health professional is essential so that your health can be monitored for you at these times.

for precisely this reason. As a result, it's essential that you perform regular blood glucose tests so that you can adjust your insulin according to the patterns of your results. By adjusting your doses properly you will be able to eat different foods and amounts and avoid hypos and a raised blood glucose level (for more information on adjusting insulin doses see pp.90–95).

From time to time you may need to try different insulins, devices, and testing kits to find those that really suit you. New injection devices and glucose testing meters are being introduced all the time – if you choose equipment that you like using, you're far more likely to want to look after your diabetes. Talk to your health professional about the choices available to you.

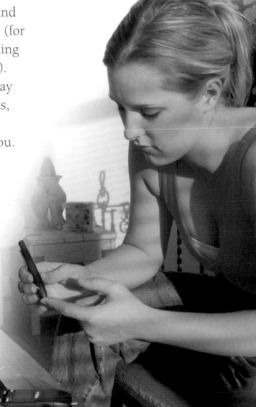

TESTING YOUR BLOOD GLUCOSE
Tests don't have to be obvious or time-consuming. Discreet pen-like devices and compact meters that give quick results are widely available.

Try different ways of looking after your diabetes to find a routine that suits you better, but avoid changing too often or too much at once. Don't try a new insulin every week, for example, or change your insulin dose, testing routine, and eating pattern all in the same week. Decide on a specific aspect of your diabetes you would like improve or change, and tackle this first before working on another aspect.

If you have Type 1 diabetes, there is one experiment you should never try: stopping your insulin completely – you can't live without it.

Dealing with hypos

If you're trying to keep your diabetes well controlled, you will have a hypo from time to time. You may feel tempted to keep your blood glucose level higher than the normal range to avoid hypos, but this isn't a good idea because it will put you at risk of complications later. Make sure you carry some form of glucose and identification at all times. If you start to get hypo symptoms, take action straight away (see pp.102–109 for more information on hypos and their treatment).

Getting on with your life

There is very little you can't do when you have diabetes. There are very few career options that are not open to you (see pp.118–119), so you can do just about any course of study or type of work. You can also take part in almost any sport. Regular physical activity is especially good for you if you have diabetes, because it helps your insulin to work efficiently, which can mean you need smaller doses. You can also drive if you want to, although there are some regulations and precautions to be aware of before you take to the road (see pp.120–122).

JOINING IN
Your diabetes won't affect your ability on the sports field or running track – but you'll need to balance your food intake and insulin so that you can perform at maximum capacity.

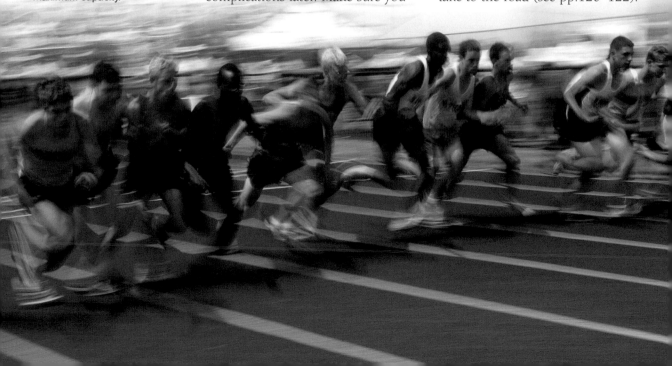

Whether you go on a school or college trip, participate in a competitive sport, work a night shift, or take an exam, your diabetes will always need some attention. When being physically active, for example, you will need to get the balance right between your food and your insulin, so you can perform at your best (see pp.56–59).

From time to time you will be unwell and because illness affects your diabetes, you'll need to know what to do about it. Your blood glucose level might be quite difficult to control because your body is fighting illness, and you might also be unable to eat and drink as normal (see pp.130–133).

Taking exams

Exams can be stressful and stress often has an effect on your blood glucose control because the hormones you produce when you are stressed – adrenaline and cortisol – make your insulin less effective (in the same way as when you are ill or during adolescence). Occasionally, stress has the opposite effect and makes you more prone to hypos. Your routine can be different while you are taking exams, too, so you may not be able to eat at your usual times.

During exam time, therefore, you need to keep a close watch on your blood glucose level by doing a few extra tests each day and changing your insulin doses when you need to. You also need to be prepared with plenty of hypo treatments, such as glucose tablets or a glucose drink,

and make sure the invigilators know that you may need to eat something during an exam. If you feel hypo in an exam, act on it straight away before it affects your concentration too much.

Drinking alcohol

Alcohol isn't banned when you have diabetes but it can affect you more severely. If you drink a lot and you have a hypo, you won't be able to recover normally because your body will be so busy processing the alcohol that it will be unable to replace the glucose in your blood. As a result, you could have a severe hypo – which can be dangerous, particularly if it happens when you are asleep at night after drinking a great deal during the evening.

For this reason it's very important to check your blood glucose level before you go to bed if you have been drinking alcohol. Aim for a blood glucose level that is 3–4 millimoles per litre above your usual bedtime level, which may mean you need a bigger bedtime snack than usual – a hypo can happen hours after you've stopped drinking.

It's also important to remember that hypoglycaemia and being drunk have similar symptoms, so other people may think you are drunk rather than hypo, especially if they smell alcohol on your breath. Be as responsible as you can about drinking and take the precaution of telling friends about hypos and

Practical tips

DRINKING ALCOHOL SAFELY

- Eat a proper carbohydrate-containing meal before you go out drinking.
- If you can't eat before you go out, make sure you have snacks that contain carbohydrate, such as sandwiches or crisps, while you are drinking.
- Carry glucose – in drink or tablet form – with you, in case you become hypo unexpectedly.
- If you're driving, don't drink any alcohol at all.

If you drink a lot and you have a hypo, you won't be able to recover normally because your body will be so busy processing the alcohol…

how to treat them should you get into trouble. (For more about drinking alcohol, see pp.38–40.)

Smoking

Having diabetes puts you at risk of circulatory problems, and this risk increases if you smoke. It is easy to say "don't smoke" but you may already have started or find it hard to resist when you are offered cigarettes by your friends. It is very important to know the following facts:
- Nicotine is highly addictive, which means that if you start smoking you'll find it difficult to stop.
- You can get help to stop smoking from national and local services and helplines, or ask your health professional for support and advice.
- Smoking increases your chances of having a heart attack, stroke, or amputation in the future because of the combined effects of smoking and diabetes on your blood vessels.

Recreational drugs

Taking recreational drugs is not a good idea when you have diabetes. Drugs can affect your concentration and your ability to look after yourself properly: you might forget to eat, eat too much, or forget to take your insulin. If you are with people who are taking drugs, they will not be able to help you if you need it. It's true that this could also happen if you don't have diabetes – but when you do have it, the chances of problems occurring are far greater.

If you decide that you are going to take any drug, you have to know exactly what you are taking, how it will affect your capability to look after your diabetes and what to do to keep yourself safe. Ask yourself the following questions:
- What effect will the drug have and for how long?
- What will happen if I take the drug and then have a hypo or forget to take my insulin?
- Who will notice or be able to help me if I become unconscious?
- Am I likely to become addicted to this drug or its effects?
- What can I do to make sure that I stay safe?

Common drugs you might be offered or choose to try include cannabis, LSD, magic mushrooms, ecstasy, speed, and cocaine. All of these drugs impair your coordination and awareness. Before taking any of these drugs, make sure you know what their effects are and how this could affect your health and your diabetes control.

■ **CANNABIS** Smoking a joint may make you feel more relaxed at the time, but it can also make you feel jittery and

---

My experience

"I remember taking LSD one day and relying on a friend to remind me to check my blood glucose and make sure I was okay. With marijuana, I'd get the munchies at 3 or 4am." JOE

COMMENT Joe describes how taking drugs as a young adult meant that he was unable to care for his diabetes properly, and had to rely on others or suffer the consequences, such as a high blood glucose level after snacking during the early hours of the morning.

uncomfortable. If you take cannabis it is easy to lose track of time, and to forget to take your insulin or look after your diabetes. It can also make you feel extremely hungry, so you might find yourself eating large amounts of high-fat and carbohydrate-rich food. If you have forgotten your insulin as well, you could end up with a seriously high blood glucose level.

■ **HALLUCINOGENICS** These drugs, which include LSD and magic mushrooms, send you on a "trip" – they make you feel as though you are in another world, with vivid images and experiences. A trip can be very frightening, and you will lose track of time as well as control of your actions and thoughts. This will make it very difficult for you to do anything to look after yourself and your diabetes.

■ **UPPERS** Drugs like ecstasy, speed, and cocaine give you what feels like boundless energy and confidence, and help you dance all night if you want to, which means that you use up a lot of energy. They can also make you very dehydrated, which can be aggravated by drinking alcohol. The combination of using energy and being dehydrated can cause severe hypoglycaemia. It's important to counteract a low blood glucose level by eating additional food and drinking extra non-alcoholic drinks. It's worth remembering, though, that you might not feel at all hungry under the influence of uppers.

Q I've been told that I can't get pregnant because I have diabetes. Does this mean I don't need contraception?

A No – you are just as likely to get pregnant when you have diabetes as anyone else. And don't believe anyone who tells you that you can't get pregnant the first time you have sex either – this is completely untrue. If you want to find out more about contraception and safe sex, your health professional will be able to advise you.

Sex and relationships

It is up to you when or if you tell a new partner about your diabetes, but if you're in a sexual relationship it may be important to do so. Because sex is a form of physical activity, it could cause you to have a hypo, either at the time or some hours later. You may need to tell your partner about this possibility and keep some glucose within reach.

If you are a woman, contraception is particularly important. Unless you are actively planning to become pregnant, either you or your partner needs to use a reliable form of contraception to prevent you from becoming pregnant by accident (see p.127).

To have a successful pregnancy when you have diabetes means that you need to prepare very carefully, and getting pregnant when your diabetes control is not very good can affect your baby's development (see pp.138–141). For more information about diabetes, sex, and relationships, see pp.126–127.

It's up to you when or if you tell a new partner about your diabetes, but if you're in a sexual relationship it may be important to do so.

Your true friends will be genuinely interested in you and your diabetes and will realize that it doesn't change who you are.

Moving away from home

Leaving home involves a complete change of routine and responsibility so it can be both exciting and slightly worrying. You will have to make all the decisions about how you manage your diabetes. You might be delighted to have your freedom, but it is important to remember the following points if you are going to live independently.

- You will be responsible for putting food in your cupboards. Make sure you have enough carbohydrate foods and hypo treatments for when you need them.
- Keep hypo treatments in your room as well as in the kitchen, especially if you share a kitchen. Your hypo supplies need to be available to you, not your flatmates!
- You should tell a friend you see regularly about your diabetes and how to treat a hypo, maybe with glucagon (see pp.106–109), in case you cannot treat it yourself.
- If you move to a new area, you'll need to register with a doctor, although you may be advised to keep your diabetes care in your home town until you move away permanently. Universities usually have on-site health centres, where you can get prescriptions and care if you are unwell. If you are working, you will need someone to contact if you're ill or you can't manage your diabetes for any reason.
- If you become ill, particularly with sickness and diarrhoea, it's important to get medical help sooner rather than later, to prevent diabetic ketoacidosis (see p.113).
- All your prescriptions are free when you take insulin or tablets, so make sure you get an exemption certificate from your doctor or pharmacist.

Talking to other people

Most people, including your potential partners, won't know much about what having diabetes means, and some people, including friends and work colleagues might have out-of-date or confused ideas about it. When other people don't understand, it can be frustrating to talk to them about diabetes, but at least one friend or colleague with whom you spend time should know something about your diabetes and how to help you if you need it.

Your diabetes is just that – yours. In general, it's up to you who you tell and what you say. What won't help, however, is to pretend you haven't got diabetes at all. It can come as quite a shock to other people if you suddenly have a hypo and they don't

Q My parents insist I come home for meals and at injection times. I hate having to rush back when I'm out – what can I do?

A If you plan your mealtimes and/or carry food with you and you take your insulin pen, it won't be necessary to be at home for meals or injections. If your parents can be sure that you'll eat and inject your insulin responsibly, they should give you a bit more freedom.

know what to do. Your family, some friends, and perhaps your colleagues or main teachers or tutors at school or college will all need to know about your diabetes so that they can help and support you when necessary.

Talking to your parents

Your parents or carers might question you about whether you've done your tests or injections and be concerned about what you're eating and drinking. You might feel like they are nagging, but usually they are just worried and trying to help you. It's a good idea to find a system that you are all happy with – and that doesn't create family tension. You may need to sit and talk calmly for a while before you come to an agreement.

Talking to your friends

If you prefer not to talk about your diabetes much, choose the person you confide in carefully and work out in advance what you are going to say. If you haven't told your friends, or you have recently been diagnosed, you might worry that they will think differently about you, especially as your treatment involves blood tests and injections. But you won't know how they will react until you tell them.

As with anything unfamiliar or surprising, it may take people a little time to get used to what you need to do to look after yourself, but after a while they'll just accept it.

If you feel that your friends respond negatively to your having diabetes, it's worth remembering

My experience

"I tell people about my diabetes because I know what I'm capable of and if they can't deal with it, then they have the problem, not me!" JANE

COMMENT You aren't responsible for other people's thoughts about your diabetes and as you feel more confident about your ability to deal with the condition, you will learn to ignore unhelpful comments.

that some people laugh at or make fun of others when they are unsure or even worried about a situation themselves. Your true friends will be genuinely interested in you and your diabetes and will realize that having diabetes doesn't change the person you are. However, if you are having to put up with a lot of hassle from other people at school or work, it's very important to report it to your teacher or employer.

CONFIDING IN FRIENDS
Some people with diabetes talk about it to just one or two close friends; others feel relaxed telling more. Who and how many people you decide to talk to about diabetes is entirely your decision.

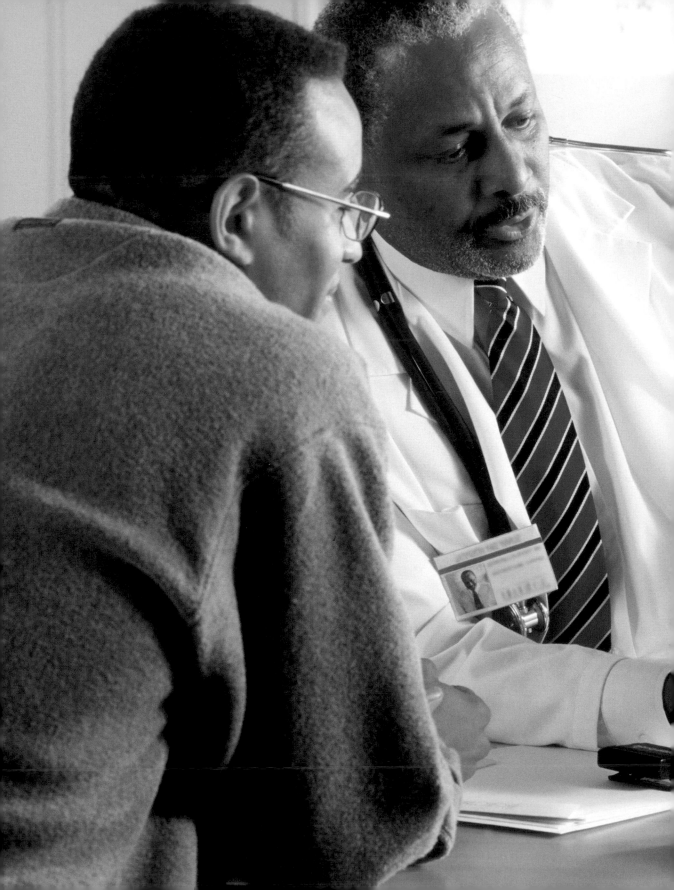

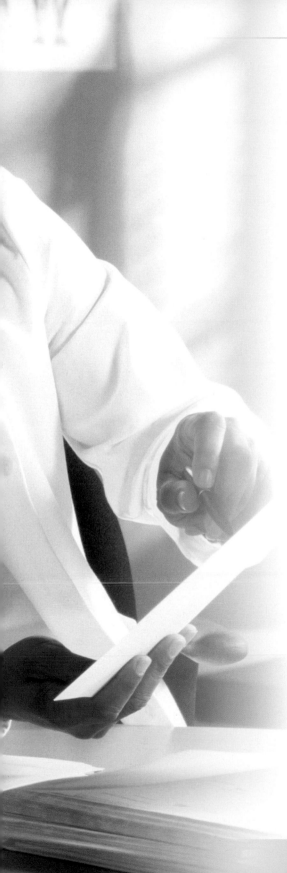

Possible long-term complications

Managing diabetes requires effort and discipline every day. You may feel unable to cope from time to time and this can develop into depression. Knowing how to deal with such feelings and what kind of help is available is important.

Having diabetes over a period of years causes physical damage to your blood vessels and nerves. Complications resulting from this damage can affect your eyes, kidneys, feet, and heart – as well as other conditions, such as sexual difficulties.

You can take practical steps to reduce your risk of developing complications, for example by keeping your blood glucose level in the recommended range; maintaining a healthy weight; eating healthily; being physically active; taking your medication regularly; and attending your review and other appointments.

Being aware of the signs of complications enables you to catch any problems early, and if you do develop complications, it is useful to know what treatment is available and what your future holds.

Depression

Depression is common in people with diabetes, partly due to the constant pressure of managing the condition and partly because of the future or current threat of long-term complications. Feeling depressed can stop you looking after yourself. This is why it's important to recognize the symptoms early and prevent things from getting worse. If you are depressed, you may benefit from counselling and/or antidepressant medication.

Around one in five people who have diabetes suffers from depression.

Understanding depression

Although depression isn't a direct complication of diabetes in the way that, for example, kidney problems (see pp.196–199) are, depression is very common in people with diabetes. Around one in five people who have diabetes suffers from depression.

Depression can be problematic if you have diabetes because when you are depressed you often feel tired and unmotivated and this can prevent you from testing your blood glucose regularly, eating food at the right time, or taking your tablets and insulin properly. If you are very depressed, you may believe that there is no point in looking after yourself.

If you think you may be vulnerable to depression, there are various steps you can take to prevent it or lessen its effects. There are also treatments available, including counselling, antidepressant medication, or a combination of both.

Causes

When you have diabetes, you may feel depressed because:
- You have just been diagnosed and you are worried or afraid of the effect diabetes will have on your life.
- You are tired of having to deal with your diabetes every day.
- You feel that your diabetes is out of your control, perhaps because your actions don't seem to be having any effect.
- You need to undergo a major change in your treatment, from tablets to insulin, for example.
- You have been told that you have signs of the long-term complications of diabetes.
- You are suffering from the advanced complications of diabetes.

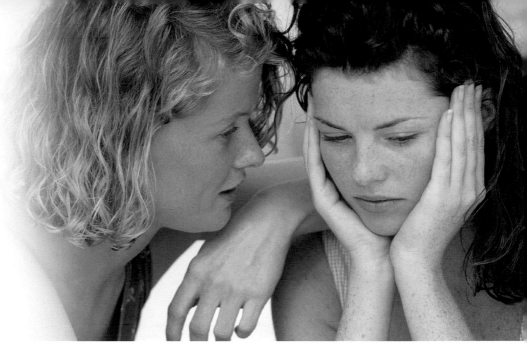

TALKING TO SOMEONE
If you are feeling low, you may find it helpful to share your feelings, either with someone you know or a professional counsellor; face-to-face or on the telephone. Talking about your feelings can help you to come to terms with them.

Alternatively, you may be depressed about something unrelated to your diabetes, such as a bereavement or the break-up of relationship. In these situations, your diabetes can contribute to your depression because it can seem like an additional burden that you don't have the energy to cope with.

Symptoms and diagnosis

There is a difference between temporarily feeling sad and depression. In the first case, your feelings are short-lived and tend not to have a major impact on your everyday life. When you are depressed, however, feelings of despair and sadness can become so dominant that you no longer feel motivated to continue with your usual activities. You may have a combination of emotional and physical symptoms and changes in your thinking, such as:

- Feelings of sadness, pessimism, or hopelessness.
- Loss of interest in your usual activities and relationships.
- Crying spells.
- Sleep disturbances.
- Loss of appetite.
- Worrying about small things.
- Fatigue, apathy, and lack of energy.
- Difficulty concentrating.
- Lack of motivation.

Your health professional can help you consider how much impact any of the above symptoms are having on your life and whether you need help to deal with them.

My experience

"When I was 14 I became very withdrawn and stopped eating. A health professional diagnosed acute depression as a result of the psychological impact of living with diabetes." SOPHIE

COMMENT Being diagnosed with diabetes can have a dramatic effect on your mind as well as your body. You may need to take more time than you think you need, in order to come to terms with the diagnosis of diabetes and its impact on your life.

My experience

"When I've been depressed my diabetes has taken a back seat because I've had no energy. I've made some rash decisions about adjusting my insulin, so my glucose has gone very high or low." SHELLEY

COMMENT A fluctuating blood glucose level can make you feel unwell and add to your depression. Acknowledging how you feel and seeking help will enable you to get back on track with your diabetes treatment.

Practical tips

DEALING WITH NEGATIVE FEELINGS

- Talk to someone – or even out loud to yourself. Simply acknowledging your feelings can be helpful.

- Take some form of regular physical activity – go for a walk, swim, or cycle ride, for example.

- Avoid putting pressure on yourself to do all the things you normally do – take time out from your busy schedule.

- Set yourself small achievable goals each day.

Prevention and treatment

Activities that bolster your sense of self-esteem can help to prevent depression. For some people, this may mean regular social contact with friends and family, for others it could mean time alone pursuing an enjoyable hobby – find out what works for you. Being physically active (see pp.52–59) has a positive effect on preventing or dealing with depression because it increases the level of mood-enhancing chemicals in your brain. It can also improve your diabetes control by helping your body to use insulin more effectively.

If your negative feelings are related to your diabetes, one of the most effective ways to overcome this is to learn as much as you can about diabetes management and put what you've learned into practice. If you feel in control of your diabetes, you can reassure yourself that you are doing your best to prevent long-term complications.

If, on the other hand, your blood glucose level is erratic and you are prone to hypos or a constantly raised blood glucose level, you are more likely to feel negative about your diabetes. If you can't control your diabetes in a way that allows you to feel confident about what you are doing, ask your health professional for advice.

Identifying that you are feeling low or not coping is important so that you can take action. You may feel as though you are failing or out of control if you admit to feelings of depression, and this can stop you getting the treatment you need.

When you first start to feel low, talking to your partner or a friend or family member can help you to explore what you are going through. It is important to choose someone who allows you to talk and listens impartially, without giving you advice. Talking about depression may be the first time that your feelings become real to you, and another person's advice or opinion may not be useful at this point. Don't be afraid to ask someone just to listen.

If you feel that your depression is getting in the way of your life and particularly if it is stopping you from managing your diabetes, it's a good idea to talk to a health professional. If you find it hard to talk about your feelings, taking a partner, friend, or family member to a consultation may help. Your health professional may recommend counselling or antidepressant tablets or both.

Even if you are feeling very depressed and unmotivated, keeping your diabetes treatment going is still worthwhile. However, you might decide to set realistic goals about how much of your diabetes care you feel able to achieve, for example you might take your tablets eight or nine times out of ten or test your blood glucose once or twice a day instead of several times.

■ **COUNSELLING** Talking to a trained counsellor about your depression can help you to develop better coping strategies or a more positive way of thinking. Your health professional can refer you for counselling or you may wish to find your own counsellor. Counselling may be one-to-one or group-based and it's important that you feel comfortable with the situation as well as with your counsellor – you should feel that you can relate to him or her.

Your counsellor may use a variety of methods to help you. This will depend on how you are coping emotionally, how anxious you are, and how much your depression is getting in the way of your daily life. For example, you may need help in coping with practical daily activities or you may need to explore the deep emotions you have about diabetes or other aspects of your life. By the time you seek help, you may have been struggling with negative feelings for months or even years, and the issues that arise can take a while to address.

Whatever method your counsellor uses, it will help you explore and start to deal with the factors that are causing your depression.

■ **ANTIDEPRESSANTS** Although antidepressants don't take away the underlying reasons for your depression, they can help you to cope more effectively. Most antidepressants work by increasing the levels of one or two chemicals in the brain: serotonin and noradrenaline. There are a variety of antidepressants available, most of which take several weeks to reach their peak effect – this means that you do not start to feel different immediately. You should expect to take antidepressants for a period of at least six months – stopping sooner can mean that your depression is likely to return. The main classes of antidepressants are:

• Tricyclic antidepressants, such as amitriptyline; these work by preventing the reabsorption and breakdown of serotonin and noradrenaline.

• Selective serotonin reuptake inhibitors (SSRIs), such as fluoxetine; these work by preventing the reabsorption and breakdown of serotonin.

• Monoamine oxidase inhibitors (MAOIs), such as phenelzine; these work by blocking the activity of an enzyme that can destroy serotonin and noradrenaline.

Outlook

It takes time to fully recover from depression and the condition can recur. You might still harbour negative feelings for months or even years after a bout of acute depression. Identifying and acting on any symptoms early can help to prevent depression from taking over your life.

Myth OR TRUTH?

MYTH
Depression is always triggered by something.

TRUTH
Tragedy or difficulties can lead to depression, but it can also occur when there is no obvious reason to be sad or negative. Dealing with diabetes every day can cause or contribute to depression, and at times you may need help to cope.

Eye conditions

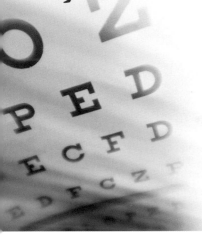

If you have diabetes, over a period of years the blood vessels at the back of your eyes can become damaged. This is known as retinopathy and can, at worst, lead to loss of sight if untreated. Annual eye examinations are vital to detect and treat problems early, and good diabetes control can prevent the condition from becoming severe enough to affect vision. Cataracts are also more common if you have diabetes and should be monitored and treated to prevent them from affecting your sight.

Retinopathy

The retina is the light-sensitive area at the back of the eye. It receives light, which the optic nerve transmits to the brain where it is interpreted as a visual image. To function properly, the retina needs a plentiful supply of blood, supplied by a network of small blood vessels.

If you have had diabetes for a long time, your eyes are vulnerable to retinopathy, which is characterized by progressive damage to these blood vessels. Retinopathy can affect one or both eyes.

■ **BACKGROUND RETINOPATHY** During the early stage of retinopathy, known as background retinopathy, blood vessels in the retina bulge and leak blood. On examination of the retina these bulges, known as microaneurysms, can be seen as small red dots. Other signs of background retinopathy are yellowish spots, known as exudates (consisting of lipoprotein – fat and protein – from leaked blood plasma), and white areas known as "cotton wool spots" in which blood vessels have closed down and stopped supplying the retina with blood. Most people who have had Type 1 diabetes for 20 years will have some background retinopathy. Background retinopathy does not necessarily progress further.

■ **PREPROLIFERATIVE RETINOPATHY** The next stage of retinopathy is known as preproliferative retinopathy. This is a

THE STRUCTURE OF THE EYE
When light enters the eye it is focused by the cornea and the lens on the retina at the back of the eye. Impulses are transmitted via the optic nerve to the brain where a visual image forms. The most sensitive area of the retina is the macula, which contains hundreds of densely packed nerve endings.

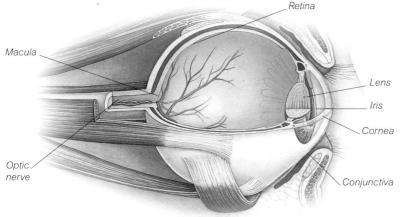

Retina

Macula

Lens

Iris

Cornea

Optic nerve

Conjunctiva

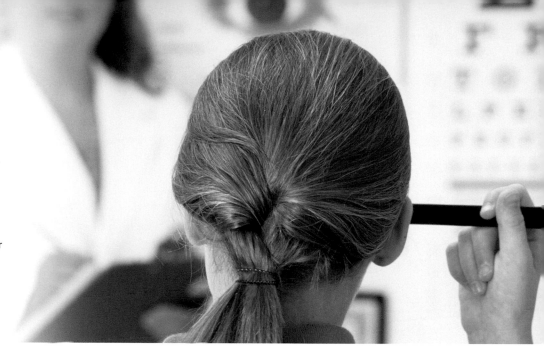

sign that damage to your eye is progressing. During an eye test, many microaneurysms, exudates, and cotton wool spots can be seen. Also, new blood vessels start to form to replace those that have closed down. These new vessels are fragile and, as a result, are prone to leaking and bleeding.

■ **PROLIFERATIVE RETINOPATHY** If preproliferative retinopathy is not treated, more fragile blood vessels form – often on top of your existing blood vessels – and this is described as proliferative retinopathy. The new blood vessels can sometimes bleed into the eye, causing reduced vision.

Causes

Retinopathy can result from a blood glucose level that has been consistently high for a period of years (although retinopathy tends to develop earlier than other long-term complications). High blood pressure can also be a contributing factor. If you have retinopathy and you become pregnant, this can cause the disease to progress more rapidly than it would normally. Also, during pregnancy, previously undiagnosed retinopathy can become

Q **What are my chances of developing retinopathy?**

A Your chance of developing retinopathy increases the longer you have diabetes. If you have had diabetes for 10 years, you have around a 50 per cent chance of having retinopathy; if you have had diabetes for 20 years, you are almost certain to have background retinopathy. This does not automatically mean that your vision is affected or that it will get worse, it may just mean that there are early signs of damage to your retinal blood vessels. If you have Type 2 diabetes, retinopathy may happen on a shorter timescale than this because it may have started to develop before you were diagnosed with diabetes. With treatment, you can stop retinopathy progressing to a stage at which your eyesight is impaired.

If you have had diabetes for a long time, your eyes are vulnerable to retinopathy.

OPHTHALMOSCOPY
The backs of your eyes are examined directly, using a hand-held ophthalmoscope, or indirectly, as shown here, using a fixed ophthalmoscope (or slit lamp).

apparent for the first time, so your eyes will be monitored more frequently during pregnancy.

Symptoms and diagnosis

Retinopathy develops gradually over years and is symptomless until the third stage (proliferative retinopathy) when vision starts to be affected. In severe cases, the complications of retinopathy (see right) may cause partial or complete sight loss. You should have an eye test to screen for retinopathy at least once a year. If you already have signs of retinopathy or you are pregnant, you are asked to have eye tests every few months. The following tests are used in the diagnosis of retinopathy.

■ **VISUAL ACUITY** This consists of reading rows of letters of diminishing size on a chart known as a Snellen chart. You stand a measured distance away and read the letters aloud, first with one eye covered and then the other. If you use spectacles, you are asked to read the chart while wearing them or to read the letters through a pinhole to see if your detailed vision has changed. If you are unable to read as many lines as at your previous eye test, retinopathy will be suspected and you will have further tests.

■ **RETINAL PHOTOGRAPHY** Your pupils are usually dilated with eye drops (unless you have a condition known as glaucoma) so that your retina can be viewed clearly. Then a digital or polaroid photograph of your retina is taken and inspected for signs of retinopathy. The advantage of digital photography is that images from consecutive eye tests can be stored electronically, or in your medical notes, making them readily available for review and comparison.

■ **OPHTHALMOSCOPY** As with retinal photography, your pupils are dilated with eye drops, then your retina is examined using one of two viewing devices: a handheld ophthalmoscope or a fixed ophthalmoscope (also known as a slit lamp). This is done in a very dark room by someone trained in ophthalmoscopy. This examination may be performed in addition to or instead of retinal photography to detect the signs of retinopathy.

■ **FLUORESCEIN ANGIOGRAPHY** A dye that is injected into a vein in your arm travels to the blood vessels in your eye. Your retina is then examined under X-ray. Fluorescein angiography is a specialized technique that isn't

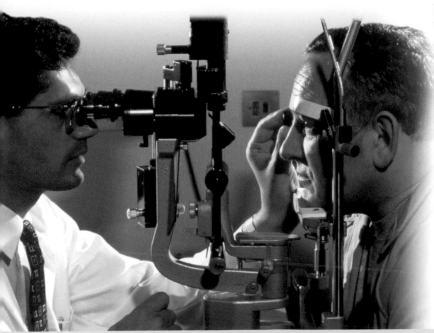

part of a routine eye test. It may be carried out if you have advanced retinopathy and it is necessary to establish the exact area of the retina that requires laser treatment.

Complications of retinopathy

The following complications of retinopathy can cause severe visual impairment and sight loss. However, all of them can be avoided if retinopathy is detected and treated from an early stage.

■ **MACULOPATHY** The macula is a central region of the retina that plays a critical role in vision. Retinopathy around the macula – known as maculopathy – may threaten your eyesight. It is more common if you have Type 2 diabetes. There are three types of maculopathy.

● Ischaemic maculopathy: small blood vessels are damaged and no longer supply blood to the macula.

● Exudative maculopathy: deposits of lipoprotein accumulate around the macula.

● Macular oedema: fluid leaks from your blood vessels and gathers around the macula.

■ **VITREOUS HAEMORRHAGE** If you have proliferative retinopathy and a large amount of bleeding takes place from the new, fragile blood vessels that have formed in your retina, this is known as a vitreous haemorrhage. You may suddenly lose a large part of your vision, although this is temporary and the blood is gradually reabsorbed.

■ **RETINAL DETACHMENT** After a vitreous haemorrhage, the blood vessels in your retina form a web that can contract and cause your retina to tear or detach from its base. Retinal detachment may happen a few weeks after a vitreous haemorrhage and can cause permanent damage to your vision.

■ **RUBEOTIC GLAUCOMA** If you have proliferative retinopathy and the new blood vessels in your eye start to grow around your iris, this causes a painful condition known as rubeotic glaucoma. This can cause visual impairment.

Prevention and treatment

The best way to prevent retinopathy from developing or progressing is good long-term blood glucose control, and, if you have high blood blood pressure, managing this correctly (see pp.206–208). It is also important to attend your appointments for eye examinations. If you have retinopathy and a high blood glucose level that suddenly falls because you have started exerting tighter control over your diabetes, your retinopathy may worsen due to changes in blood vessel structure. Improving your blood glucose level over a period of months rather than weeks can prevent this.

Treatment of retinopathy depends on how advanced the condition is. In the early stages of retinopathy (background retinopathy), you don't need any treatment, but your eyes need to be examined for any signs of deterioration every six months.

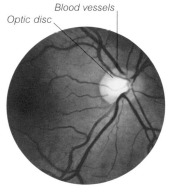

Blood vessels
Optic disc

Healthy retina

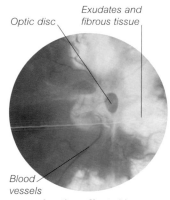

Exudates and fibrous tissue
Optic disc
Blood vessels

A retina affected by proliferative retinopathy

THE RETINA
The ophthalmoscope's view of a healthy retina shows a network of healthy blood vessels extending from the optic nerve. In the retina affected by proliferative retinopathy, blood supply is greatly impeded and the retina is partially covered by fatty exudates and fibrous tissue.

"Twelve years ago, after 30 years of diabetes, I developed retinopathy and had haemorrhages in both my eyes. It was a big shock. I work much harder to control my diabetes now." JOE

COMMENT If you have retinopathy that has been treated satisfactorily or you are in the early stages of retinopathy, maintaining good control of your blood glucose level and blood pressure can prevent problems recurring in the future or progressing to the next stage.

If you receive treatment for retinopathy and your condition stabilizes, the amount of time between your eye examinations can gradually increase.

If you have a later stage of retinopathy (preproliferative or proliferative retinopathy), you are given laser treatment. It is not necessary to be admitted to hospital for this; the treatment can be performed at a specialist outpatient clinic. The procedure consists of directing laser beams at the damaged areas of your retina, in order to destroy the fragile blood vessels that have formed. If you need a lot of laser treatment, this might take place over several visits. Laser treatment carried out during pregnancy does not harm your unborn baby.

Laser treatment is also used to treat maculopathy (with the exception of ischaemic maculopathy, which cannot be treated). You can also have laser treatment after a vitreous haemorrhage, but only after the blood has been reabsorbed by your body – it isn't possible to get a clear view of your retina before this. Laser treatment can prevent deterioration in your vision but cannot restore lost vision.

Sometimes eye surgery may be recommended to treat vitreous haemorrhage and retinal detachment.

Although surgery can help to restore quite a lot of your vision, it does not restore it completely because of the extensive damage that has already occurred to your retina. Surgery might also be used to relieve the pain of rubeotic glaucoma.

If you receive treatment for retinopathy and your condition stabilizes, the amount of time between your eye examinations can gradually increase until the point at which you only need to attend appointments every six months or yearly. If any problems develop in the future, you are referred back to your eye clinic for further investigation and treatment.

Outlook

Retinopathy can be successfully treated and complete loss of vision can be prevented by good diabetes control, regular and thorough monitoring, and prompt surgery or laser treatment.

Cataracts

If you have diabetes, you are more prone to developing cataracts, in which the lens of the eye, which is normally clear, becomes cloudy.

Causes

Cataracts occur as a result of structural changes to protein fibres within the lens. Changes in the protein fibres are a normal part of ageing – which is why people who don't have diabetes can also develop them – but they can also be caused by a blood glucose level that has been high for many years.

Symptoms and diagnosis

The cloudiness of the lens prevents sufficient light from entering the eye, resulting in a partial loss of vision. Also, bright lights may appear to have a halo. Because cataracts are progressive, they cause a gradual deterioration in vision (not complete sight loss, as light enters the eye even when cataracts are advanced). Cataracts are diagnosed using an ophthalmoscope (see p.192).

Prevention and treatment

You can reduce your risk of developing cataracts by maintaining good long-term control of your blood glucose. Cataracts can be surgically removed under local anaesthetic and you will have a new lens inserted.

Outlook

Cataracts develop slowly and may never reach the stage at which they require surgical treatment. If you have surgery, however, your vision will be completely restored.

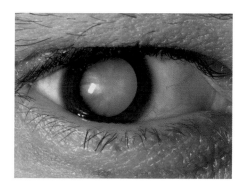

MATURE CATARACT
Changes to protein fibres in the eye cause the lens to become increasingly opaque. Over time, this causes vision to deteriorate. Cataracts can be treated successfully with surgery.

Living with reduced vision

If your vision is adversely affected by retinopathy or cataracts, making adjustments in your life will enable you to cope. You are entitled to a range of benefits and support to help you do this. To find out more, contact a national organization that works on behalf of people with reduced vision (see p.218).

Impaired vision can affect your ability to manage everyday tasks, and specifically those that are related to your diabetes. If testing your blood glucose level, taking tablets, and/or injecting yourself with insulin is difficult, ask your health professional about equipment that can make things easier; for example, a blood glucose meter that has a memory (so that someone else can read your results at a convenient time) or an insulin delivery device with a fixed dose. Hypos (see pp.102–109) can be problematic if you have impaired vision because you may not be able to see well enough to treat yourself. You can ask someone close to you for help if you find such tasks difficult or talk to your health professional if you are worried about managing your insulin dosage.

If you drive, you may need to take an eye test, including a field of vision test, to establish whether it is safe for you to continue driving. A field of vision test measures the size of your area of vision on each side (this should be at least 120 degrees).

Myth OR TRUTH?

MYTH
Blurred vision is always a sign of retinopathy.

TRUTH
Blurred vision can be a symptom of a temporarily raised blood glucose level. If your vision becomes blurred, check your blood glucose level and if it is high, take measures to correct it – you may need to adjust your tablet or insulin dosage. Your vision should correct itself up to 6 weeks after your blood glucose has improved. In this circumstance, blurred vision is not a sign of retinopathy and provided you continue to keep your blood glucose level in check, should not lead to any long-term problems.

Kidney conditions

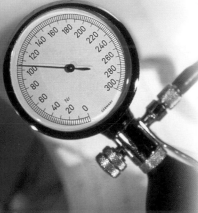

Kidney damage, which may occur when you have had diabetes for many years, is known as nephropathy. Symptoms rarely occur until the damage is extensive, so urine and blood tests are used to detect problems early. Good blood glucose and blood pressure control can prevent nephropathy progressing to a stage where large amounts of protein are lost in the urine, which can indicate kidney damage that can lead to end-stage renal failure and the need for dialysis or a kidney transplant.

THE KIDNEYS
Each kidney contains about a million mini filtering units, called nephrons, each of which contains a cluster of capillaries (glomerulus), which filter blood, and a long tube called the renal tubule, which reabsorbs beneficial substances.

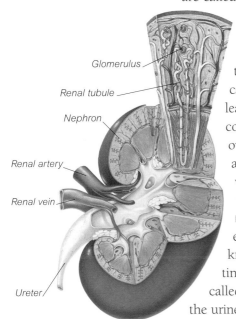

Glomerulus

Renal tubule

Nephron

Renal artery

Renal vein

Ureter

Nephropathy

The kidneys filter the blood and get rid of waste products by making urine. They also regulate the amount of fluid and salts in the body – helping to control blood pressure. The kidneys' main filtering units are called nephrons. Nephropathy, also known as renal disease, progressively reduces the kidneys' ability to function properly, which causes illness and sometimes leads to kidney failure. The condition develops slowly over a period of years, affecting about 3 in 10 people who have had diabetes for more than 15 years.

■ **MICROALBUMINURIA** In the earliest stage of nephropathy, known as microalbuminuria, tiny amounts of a protein called albumin are found in the urine. This is a sign of early kidney damage, which can be reversed with treatment.

■ **PROTEINURIA** If the condition worsens, proteinuria, which means an abnormal quantity of protein in the urine, can develop and if protein is consistently present, it means that the kidneys have sustained permanent damage. You can have proteinuria temporarily if you have a kidney or bladder infection, and the excess protein disappears when the infection clears up and is not linked to permanent kidney damage.

■ **END-STAGE RENAL FAILURE** Untreated proteinuria can lead to end-stage renal failure – the kidneys can no longer function properly and dialysis or a kidney transplant are required.

Causes

Nephropathy occurs as a result of a high blood glucose level over a period of years, which causes damage to the nephrons. High blood pressure can

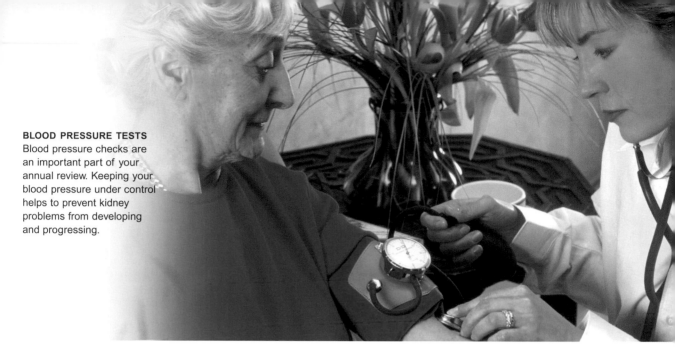

BLOOD PRESSURE TESTS
Blood pressure checks are an important part of your annual review. Keeping your blood pressure under control helps to prevent kidney problems from developing and progressing.

also cause further damage to the kidneys. The first part of the nephron to be affected is a cluster of tiny blood vessels, called the glomerulus. These blood vessels become blocked and leaky, causing protein to escape into the urine and some waste products to remain in the blood. Over time, the filtering tubule in the nephron also becomes damaged, and increasing amounts of protein are excreted in the urine.

If you have had Type 1 diabetes for 20 years, you have a 30 per cent chance of developing nephropathy. If you haven't developed nephropathy after 30 years, however, you are unlikely to do so. Less is known about Type 2 diabetes and the risk of nephropathy, but if you have Type 2 diabetes and you also have high blood pressure, or if you are of South Asian descent, your chances of developing nephropathy are significantly increased.

Symptoms and diagnosis

Microalbuminuria does not produce any symptoms, which is why your health professional will carry out urine tests once or twice a year to check for signs of early kidney damage. A single positive test for microalbuminuria does not necessarily indicate kidney damage: a urine infection can also cause levels of microalbuminuria to rise. For this reason, if a single test is positive, you will have two follow-up tests. If two out of three test results are abnormal, microalbuminuria is diagnosed.

If you develop proteinuria, your kidneys are no longer able to filter out waste products or remove excess fluids efficiently. When these build up in your body they can cause fluid retention, such as swollen ankles or legs, shortness of breath, tiredness, nausea, and itchy skin. Sometimes, however, proteinuria produces no symptoms at all. You will usually have

Myth OR TRUTH?

MYTH
Once you start to develop nephropathy, it can only get worse.

TRUTH
If nephropathy is treated at the earliest stage, when only very small amounts of protein are present in the urine, your kidneys can recover completely and function normally again. Excellent blood glucose and blood pressure control are essential to avoid further damage.

HAEMODIALYSIS AND PERITONEAL DIALYSIS

There are two forms of dialysis: haemodialysis, in which a kidney machine filters the blood, and peritoneal dialysis, also known as Continuous Ambulatory Peritoneal Dialysis (CAPD), in which the peritoneal membrane is used as a filter. The type of dialysis you have depends on your health, personal preference, and what is available locally. Your health professional will discuss your options with you.

PROCEDURE	HAEMODIALYSIS	PERITONEAL DIALYSIS
How it works	Blood is pumped by a machine through a filter attached to the side of the machine. Inside the filter, waste products and water pass from the blood into dialysis fluid, and the filtered blood returns to the body.	The peritoneal membrane surrounding the abdominal organs is used to filter blood. Dialysis fluid is infused into the peritoneal cavity via tubing attached to a catheter in the abdominal wall. It is drained out a few hours later and replaced with fresh dialysis fluid.
Preparation before starting treatment	Surgery is needed before treatment can start, to connect an artery and vein, usually in your arm, so that the dialysis machine can be connected to your circulatory system.	Surgery is needed before treatment can start, to insert a small tube called a catheter in your abdomen. The catheter can be attached to dialysis equipment.
Where dialysis is carried out	Usually at a dialysis centre, but some people are able to treat themselves at home.	At home.
Treatment duration/frequency	3–4 hours, 3 times a week.	1 hour, 4 or more times a day.
Other considerations	Haemodialysis can affect diabetes control and cause hypos, so you will need to monitor your blood glucose and adjust your treatment regularly. Other medications and changes to your food intake will be necessary.	You may need to alter the dose of any diabetes medication you take because most dialysis fluid contains glucose, which affects your blood glucose level. You will be prescribed other medications and will need to pay attention to your food intake.

If nephropathy is diagnosed, you need to bring your blood glucose under tight control.

a 24-hour urine test – this involves saving all the urine you pass over a 24-hour period in a bottle, which is sent for laboratory analysis to reveal how much protein you excrete in a day. You will also have a blood test to measure the creatinine and urea in your blood (waste products that your kidneys should excrete). Your kidneys may also be scanned using ultrasound to look for other causes of proteinuria.

The main symptoms of end-stage renal failure usually include swelling of the face, limbs, and abdomen, a greatly reduced volume of urine, severe lethargy, weight loss, headache, vomiting, and very itchy skin. Urine tests and blood tests are used to detect abnormal levels of waste products in these body fluids.

Prevention and treatment
Keeping your blood glucose and blood pressure under control are important ways in which you can prevent nephropathy from developing or progressing. If nephropathy is diagnosed, you need to bring your

blood glucose under tight control. If your blood pressure is high, this can make the condition worse, so you may be prescribed tablets to lower your blood pressure. Stopping smoking, losing weight if you need to, cutting down on salt, and eating less fat if you have high fat (lipid) levels also help to lower blood pressure. You may also be prescribed ACE (angiotensin converting enzyme) inhibitor tablets, such as ramipril or lisinopril, which help to reduce the amount of protein you lose through your kidneys, and slow the progression of the condition. You will then be monitored with regular blood pressure checks, twice-yearly blood and urine tests to check your kidney function, and twice-yearly HbA1c tests (see p.66) to check your blood glucose control.

If you develop proteinuria, you may be asked to eat less protein and cut down on foods that are high in potassium (for example, potato crisps, yeast extract, and bananas) or salt to prevent waste products from building up in your body. You will need to see a specialist dietitian for advice. Your diabetes medication may also need to be changed because some tablets, particularly metformin, should not be taken if you have nephropathy.

If you develop end-stage renal failure, the main treatment options are haemodialysis or peritoneal dialysis, both of which take over the functions of filtering waste products from the blood (see box, left). You may be offered a kidney transplant, but this is less likely to be an option if you have severe heart disease. A kidney transplant also depends upon finding a suitable organ donor, and you will need dialysis in the meantime.

If you take tablets for your diabetes, you will probably need to change to insulin injections instead. This is because your kidneys are no longer able to excrete diabetes tablets, so they will build up in your body and make you more prone to hypoglycaemia or other side effects. For the same reason, if you already take insulin, you may need smaller doses than before to control your blood glucose level. You will receive advice from a specialist dietitian about which foods are recommended and which may need to be avoided when you have renal failure. You will also need to limit your fluid intake, possibly to no more than one litre per day.

Outlook

Nephropathy can be successfully treated in the early stages, especially microalbuminuria, and tight control of your blood glucose and blood pressure can reduce your risk of developing nephropathy, slow down, or even halt its progression. If you develop end-stage renal failure, however, the damage is irreversible. You will need dialysis, or a kidney transplant if this is a suitable option for you.

HAEMODIALYSIS
If you develop end-stage renal failure, you will need dialysis or a renal transplant. Dialysis involves being connected via tubing to a machine that filters waste products from your blood.

Foot conditions

When you have diabetes, foot conditions can be caused by damage to the nerves in your legs – peripheral neuropathy – or by reduced blood flow to your feet – peripheral ischaemia. If you have either or both of these conditions, you are more prone to associated complications, such as foot ulcers, Charcot foot, and severe infections, such as gangrene. Knowing the risks, checking your feet daily, and promptly seeking help for any concerns you have can prevent problems arising.

At least once a year, you need an examination to identify whether your feet are affected by peripheral neuropathy.

Peripheral neuropathy

Damage to the nerves supplying the extremities of your body is known as peripheral neuropathy. The condition, which causes pain or loss of feeling in the toes and feet, can occur in anyone who has had diabetes for several years. If you have Type 2 diabetes, you may already have peripheral neuropathy by the time you are diagnosed with diabetes. Peripheral neuropathy may affect a small part of one foot, parts of both feet, or all of both feet. It can also affect your lower legs. Rarely, it can affect your arms and hands.

Causes

Periods of high blood glucose and high blood pressure (see pp.206–208) over months and years cause damage to nerves all over your body. The nerves supplying your feet and lower legs are very long, so if they become damaged and less efficient, these parts of your body will be affected first. In addition, your feet are particularly vulnerable because they carry your entire body weight and have a great deal of pressure on them.

Symptoms and diagnosis

Symptoms of peripheral neuropathy may include:
- A tingling, burning, or prickling sensation (you might feel pins and needles, for example).
- Short, stabbing, or burning pains, which can be very severe and often occur at night.
- Numbness or insensitivity to temperature or pain.
- Extreme sensitivity to touch (even a light touch, such as bedclothes lying on your feet at night).

You might have no symptoms at all, or you may experience symptoms and find that they change over time, because nerve damage gradually reduces the feeling in your feet. At

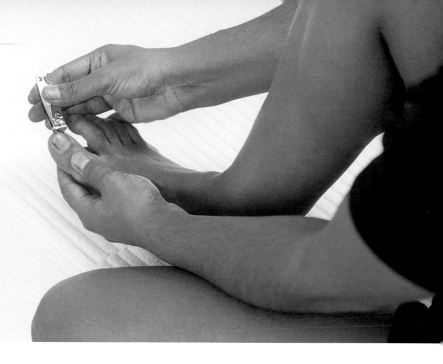

CARING FOR YOUR FEET
When you have diabetes, it is very important to have a daily routine of washing, drying, moisturizing, and checking your feet for any signs of pressure or redness. Keeping your toenails clipped is also important.

least once a year, you need an examination to identify whether your feet are affected by peripheral neuropathy. The health professional examining your feet can tell you if parts of your feet have reduced feeling. Your feet are examined for:

- Any areas of altered sensation.
- Reddened areas that suggest pressure from your shoes.
- Very dry skin.
- Hard skin (callus) beneath which ulcers (a complication of peripheral neuropathy, see pp.204–205) can form.
- Abnormal warmth.
- Wounds or open sores.
- Any deformities or change in the shape of your foot due to weakening of your foot muscles.

To assess your sensation, your health professional uses various different pieces of equipment, such as cotton wool, a sharp instrument called a neurotip, a nylon filament called a monofilament, or a vibration tuning fork to touch areas of your feet. You are asked whether you are able to feel each touch in order to identify any areas of your feet that have reduced feeling. Your health professional also checks the two pulses in each of your feet, one on the top of your foot, and the other behind your ankle bone. A faint or absent pulse may suggest another condition called peripheral ischaemia (see pp.202–204), which can occur in conjunction with neuropathy. You may also have your ankle and knee reflexes tested because peripheral neuropathy can cause muscle weakness and loss of these reflexes.

Prevention and treatment

You can prevent peripheral neuropathy or stop it from getting worse by good blood glucose control. Taking meticulous care of your feet can help to identify any problems at an early stage (see pp.128–130).

Myth OR TRUTH?

MYTH
If my feet feel fine, my diabetes can't have caused any damage to them.

TRUTH
The damage that diabetes causes happens gradually, so you won't necessarily realize that the sensation in your feet is reduced unless you ask your health professional to alert you to any problems at your annual review, and then regularly check your feet yourself.

Practical tips

CARING FOR YOUR FEET

- Check your feet daily for sores or wounds.
- Keep the area between your toes dry.
- Use an unperfumed moisturizer every day.
- Avoid wearing shoes that are too tight.
- Check your shoes for any stones or sharp objects.
- Don't put your feet directly on hot sand, radiators, or a hot-water bottle.
- Avoid using corn plasters or other dressings that contain chemicals.
- If hard skin (callus) starts to build up, have it assessed by a health professional.

If you have peripheral neuropathy, you have a higher risk of damaging your feet through everyday activities. Ask your health professional which parts of your feet have reduced sensation and where problems might develop as a result. Even if you have no soreness or discomfort, it is vital to check your feet daily for pressure areas or constant redness, which could, in time, lead to an ulcer. Talk to your health professional in advance about how to get help, so that you can act quickly if you need to.

If you have painful peripheral neuropathy, you may be prescribed tablets to help relieve the pain. You may be given antidepressants such as amitriptyline or imipramine, or anticonvulsants, such as gabapentin or carbamazepine. These have been found to be effective in reducing pain from neuropathy. If your peripheral neuropathy progresses, your pain will gradually reduce as the nerves become more damaged. This makes observation and care of your feet even more important.

Creams that you can apply to painful areas can also be helpful. Cream containing capsaicin, an extract of hot chilli peppers, is one example, although you should keep it away from open wounds and wash your hands thoroughly after using it. If bedclothes are irritating your feet and legs at night, applying a film dressing, or even clingfilm, can protect sensitive areas of your feet. You can also obtain a bed cradle to raise bedsheets away from your feet and legs.

Outlook

Peripheral neuropathy is irreversible but you can prevent it worsening by maintaining tight blood glucose control, perhaps by starting insulin injections. Complications associated with peripheral neuropathy are more likely, including foot ulcers (see pp.204–205) and Charcot foot (see p.205). Acute peripheral neuropathy is occasionally resolved by a dramatic improvement in blood glucose control.

Peripheral ischaemia

Ischaemia is a condition in which the blood supply all over your body is reduced because your arteries are narrowed. Ischaemia that affects your legs and feet is known as peripheral ischaemia and results in an insufficient supply of oxygen and nutrients to these parts of your body.

Causes of ischaemia

Peripheral ischaemia is caused by atherosclerosis, in which gradual damage takes place to the inside walls of the arteries. Risk factors for atherosclerosis, and therefore peripheral ischaemia, are smoking, a high level of cholesterol in the blood (known as hyperlipidaemia), a high-fat diet, and a high blood glucose level over a period of years.

Symptoms and diagnosis

Symptoms usually develop gradually over months or years and include:
- A cramp-like pain in your calves following exertion or, less commonly, when you are inactive.

- Cold, pale feet.
- Wounds or injuries that are slow to heal (a lack of blood flow to your feet means that wounds are deprived of the oxygen and nutrients they need to heal properly).
- Persistent foot ulcers.

You may not experience any symptoms at all, but peripheral ischaemia can be diagnosed during a foot examination as part of your annual review (see p.26). Your health professional assesses the feeling in your feet, and checks your foot pulses (faint or absent pulses are a sign of ischaemia). If your foot sensation is reduced, this suggests that you may have a condition called peripheral neuropathy (see pp.200–202), which often occurs in conjunction with peripheral ischaemia. If you are diagnosed with peripheral ischaemia, you may be referred for a number of investigations including blood tests, ultrasound scans, or special X-rays to assess how efficiently blood is flowing through your blood vessels.

Prevention and treatment

Healthy eating, regular physical activity, and stopping smoking all help to prevent peripheral ischaemia. Taking any medication you are prescribed to control blood glucose and blood pressure also reduces risk and helps to prevent peripheral ischaemia from getting worse.

If peripheral ischaemia is mild, regular checks by your health professional combined with lifestyle changes, in particular, stopping smoking, may be suggested. If the condition is severe and the blood flow to your feet is seriously reduced, you may need surgery. Affected arteries can be widened using a technique called angioplasty, in which a small balloon on the tip of a tube is passed into the artery and inflated. You may need surgery to bypass damaged blood vessels. If the blood supply to your foot is blocked and this cannot be rectified with surgery, or if your foot becomes infected and will not heal, or if gangrene (see p.205) develops, you may need an amputation of part or all of your affected foot.

CHARACTERISTICS OF FOOT CONDITIONS

Peripheral neuropathy and ischaemia cause different problems and have different characteristics. However, it is possible to have a combination of the conditions, known as neuroischaemia, which further increases your chances of developing foot problems.

PERIPHERAL NEUROPATHY	PERIPHERAL ISCHAEMIA
Warm skin.	Cool or cold skin.
Lack of feeling in foot or feet.	Normal or slightly reduced feeling.
Pink or normal colour.	Pale or blue-tinged colour.
May be painless, but pain can occur and is most severe at night.	Painful during exertion or rest at any time of day.
Normal or increased pulses in the feet.	Faint pulses in the feet, or no pulses at all.
Callused skin.	No callus.
Reduced reflexes.	Normal reflexes.
Prone to ulcers on any areas of pressure, for example, the soles of the feet.	Prone to ulcers on the sides of the feet.
Potential to develop Charcot (misshapen) foot.	Potential to develop gangrene.

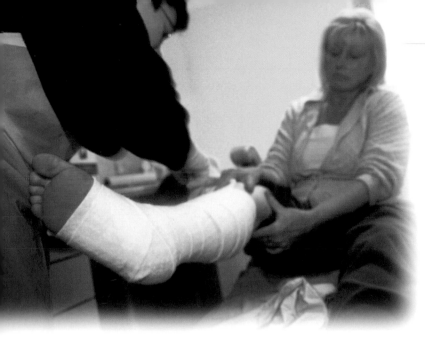

Outlook

Peripheral ischaemia is irreversible, but it can be stabilized or treated to improve blood flow. You may need some treatments, for example, bypass surgery, more than once. Making lifestyle changes to limit further blood vessel damage is important. You will always be susceptible to associated complications such as foot ulcers, Charcot foot, and gangrene.

Complications of peripheral neuropathy and ischaemia

The following complications of peripheral neuropathy and/or peripheral ischaemia can cause severe infection, foot deformity, and a loss of blood supply to your feet, which, eventually, can make amputation necessary.

■ **FOOT ULCERS** A complication of peripheral neuropathy, or ischaemia, or both, foot ulcers need immediate attention to prevent serious infection.

They are more likely to develop on the soles of your feet or on any areas of increased pressure if you have peripheral neuropathy, and on the sides of your feet if you have peripheral ischaemia. Ulcers can develop beneath a layer of callused skin, or be caused by an injury, such as walking on a sharp object, a burn, or a blister resulting from tight or rubbing footwear.

Ulcers do not always hurt, so if you can see any broken or callused skin on one or both of your feet, contact your health professional as soon as possible. In untreated ulcers, layers of skin and underlying foot tissue are gradually destroyed, creating a hole that may sometimes go as deep as your bone. If this happens, you are at risk of developing osteomyelitis (a bone infection). If you have peripheral ischaemia, there is a risk that your ulcer may become gangrenous (see p.205).

Ulcers need to heal from their deepest point under the skin outwards, so your health professional will remove skin or pus above the ulcer and clean out any dead or infected tissue inside. Your ulcer will then be dressed to protect against infection.

It is vitally important to avoid putting any pressure on your ulcer while it is healing. Walking on an ulcer can make it larger and force an infection deeper into your foot. Your health professional may put a special shoe or cast on your foot to protect it and remove pressure. You might need to wear this for up to 12 weeks to allow the ulcer to heal completely.

Your health professional will take a swab from the wound, which is analysed in a laboratory to find out whether you have an infection and which type of antibiotics will best treat it. You may be asked to take a long course of antibiotics, possibly for up to eight weeks, to ensure that your infection is controlled (you may need more than one long course of treatment). If your ulcer is severely infected, you may need to stay in hospital to take all the pressure off your ulcer and have intravenous antibiotics. If an abscess forms, you may need an operation to drain the abscess. An infection that is very deep or will not heal may mean that part of your foot needs to be amputated so that infection is prevented from spreading.

Ulcers take a very long time to heal, but once your ulcer heals, you will need to treat your foot extremely carefully to prevent it from returning – scar tissue at the site of an ulcer can break. Good blood glucose control is important if you have an ulcer or are prone to ulcers, as it reduces the chances of infection (a high blood glucose level makes your body less able to fight infection).

■ **CHARCOT FOOT** This is a complication of peripheral neuropathy, in which the bones of the feet become damaged. Your bone thickness is reduced by neuropathy and a small injury to your foot can cause the bones to quickly fracture or disintegrate. This can dislocate your foot joints. New bone forms at the site of the damage and, as a result, your foot becomes misshapen.

Early signs of Charcot foot are a hot, swollen foot that gets worse over 2–3 months, and might be painful or ache. Treating Charcot foot involves keeping the weight off affected parts of your feet, usually by wearing a cast in the short-term and specially made footwear in the longer-term. If you have Charcot foot, your foot will change shape over time, so shoes that fit you one day might not fit properly in six months' time. Wear shoes made from flexible material, such as leather, and with adjustable fastenings, such as laces, so that they can adapt to the shape of your foot as it changes. The process of new bone formation will slow and stop after a few months, but permanent deformities will remain.

■ **GANGRENE** This is a complication of peripheral ischaemia, in which an area of your foot loses its blood supply altogether. If the blood supply to any part of your foot is cut off, such as to a toe or heel, the skin turns a bluish-purple colour and then black. Once a toe or foot has developed gangrene, an amputation is necessary to prevent the gangrene spreading further. If you have had ulcers and pain in your leg for years, an amputation before gangrene develops may improve your quality of life, as it enables you to live without pain.

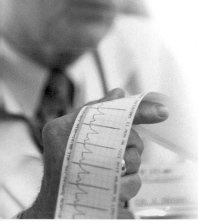

Cardiovascular conditions

Diabetes is strongly linked to high blood pressure and hyperlipidaemia, which as well as being cardiovascular (heart and circulatory) conditions in themselves, are also major risk factors for other such conditions, for example, coronary heart disease, stroke, and peripheral vascular disease. Identifying your individual risk factors and making appropriate changes to your lifestyle will help to prevent cardiovascular conditions developing.

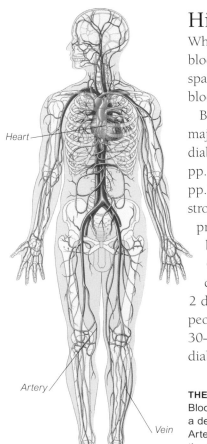

Heart

Artery

Vein

THE CARDIOVASCULAR SYSTEM
Blood is pumped by the heart through a dense network of arteries and veins. Arteries carry oxygen-rich blood from the heart to tissues all over the body. Veins carry blood back to the heart.

High blood pressure

When arteries are stiff and narrow, blood is forced through a smaller space at a high pressure – this is high blood pressure (hypertension).

Because high blood pressure is a major cause of other complications of diabetes, such as eye conditions (see pp.190–195), kidney conditions (see pp.196–199), coronary heart disease, stroke, and peripheral vascular disease, prevention and treatment of high blood pressure are essential.

Cardiovascular disease is the main cause of death in people with Type 2 diabetes. Around 10–30 per cent of people with Type 1 diabetes and 30–60 per cent of people with Type 2 diabetes have high blood pressure.

Causes

Although the link between high blood pressure and diabetes is not yet fully understood, high blood pressure is thought to be partly caused by a high level of insulin circulating in the blood due to insulin resistance in Type 2 diabetes or insulin treatment in Type 1 diabetes. As a result, blood vessels become scarred, and hard plaques form. In Type 1 diabetes, high blood pressure often occurs if your kidney function starts to deteriorate; in Type 2 diabetes it is linked with hyperlipidaemia and central body obesity. Lack of physical activity, smoking, high alcohol consumption, and stress are also risk factors.

Symptoms and diagnosis

High blood pressure rarely produces symptoms. If you have diabetes and a blood pressure of 140/80 millimetres of mercury (mmHg) or above when you are tested on several occasions,

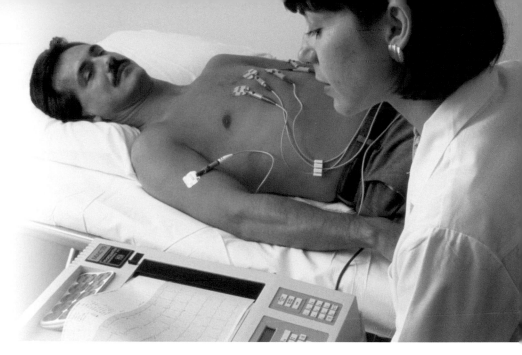

HEART MONITORING
Electrocardiography (ECG) is used to record the electrical activity of the heart and to diagnose abnormal heart rhythms or to investigate the cause of chest pain.

you are diagnosed with high blood pressure. The first figure in a blood pressure reading refers to the pressure when your heart contracts (systolic pressure), the second figure refers to when your heart relaxes between beats (diastolic pressure).

Prevention and treatment

There are very important steps you can take to prevent high blood pressure:
- Eat healthily as much as possible.
- Keep physically active.
- Stop smoking.
- Lose weight if you need to.

Maintaining good blood glucose control and keeping your alcohol consumption within normal limits also helps. If you have been diagnosed with high blood pressure, reducing your salt intake can be helpful.

If your blood pressure is high on several occasions, you will receive treatment and be reviewed every three to six months. The following

tablets are used to treat high blood pressure (you may need to take up to three different types of tablet).
- Beta-blockers, such as atenolol and oxprenolol; these work by blocking the action of adrenaline, a hormone that increases your heart rate and raises blood pressure.
- Diuretics (in low doses), such as bendroflumethiazide and indapamide; these work by decreasing fluid volume in your body and dilating your arteries.
- Angiotensin converting enzyme inhibitors (ACE inhibitors) such as ramipril and enalapril; these work by dilating your arteries.
- Calcium-channel blockers, such as amlodipine and nifedipine; these work by blocking the mechanism that causes your arteries to constrict.

Outlook

If your blood pressure is maintained at 140/80 mmHg or below, either by changes in your lifestyle or by taking

Practical tips

STOPPING SMOKING SUCCESSFULLY

- Try nicotine skin patches or nicotine chewing gum.
- Attend a stopping smoking clinic.
- Change your routine and associations. For example, if you always smoke after a meal, go for a walk after meals instead.
- Socialize in places where you can't smoke, such as the cinema instead of a bar, or the non-smoking section of a restaurant.
- If you feel you can't stop completely, start by cutting down to one or two cigarettes a day.

tablets, this greatly reduces your risk of developing coronary heart disease, stroke, peripheral vascular disease, and eye and kidney conditions.

Hyperlipidaemia

An abnormally high level of fats (lipids) in the blood, referred to as hyperlipidaemia, is a major cause of coronary heart disease, stroke, and peripheral artery disease. It is more common in people with Type 2 diabetes. If you have Type 1 diabetes, you are likely to have normal levels of fats in the blood unless there is another reason for them to be raised.

Causes

The link between diabetes and hyperlipidaemia isn't fully understood, but the abnormally high level of insulin caused by insulin resistance in Type 2 diabetes is thought to be partly responsible. If you have Type 2 diabetes, you are more likely to develop the condition if you are obese and have high blood pressure.

Other general risk factors in either Type 1 or Type 2 diabetes include a high-fat diet, inactivity, smoking, obesity, an underactive thyroid gland, and a high blood glucose level over years. A high alcohol intake and/or a family history of hyperlipidaemia are also contributing factors.

Symptoms and diagnosis

Hyperlipidaemia rarely produces symptoms. At your annual review (see p.26) you have a blood test to measure cholesterol. If the result is high, you are given healthy eating advice. You may be offered more blood tests to find out the levels of other lipids: triglycerides, low-density lipoprotein (LDL), and high-density lipoprotein (HDL). See chart.

Prevention and treatment

There is much you can do to prevent hyperlipidaemia: eating healthily – in particular avoiding saturated fats (see p.36) – becoming more physically active, and losing weight are very important. Good diabetes control and reducing a high alcohol intake can also help. Treatment consists of tablets; which type you need depends on your blood fat level:

● Statins, such as simvastatin and pravastatin; these work by preventing cholesterol production.
● Fibrates, such as bezafibrate and ciprofibrate; these work by reducing the production of triglycerides.

Your blood lipid levels may be tested every three to six months to assess whether treatment is working.

HEALTHY LEVELS OF FATS IN THE BLOOD

High levels of some fats (lipids) in the blood – and low levels of others – increase your risk of coronary heart disease. If you have a blood test to check your lipid levels, these are the results that you need to aim for to keep your heart and blood vessels healthy.

TYPE OF FAT	HEALTHY LEVEL
Cholesterol	Below 4.0 millimoles per litre
Triglycerides	Below 1.7 millimoles per litre
LDL cholesterol	Below 2.0 millimoles per litre
HDL cholesterol	Above 1.0 millimoles per litre (men) Above 1.2 millimoles per litre (women)

Outlook

If your blood lipid levels remain healthy due to changes in your lifestyle or to taking tablets, your risk of developing coronary heart disease, stroke, and peripheral vascular disease is significantly reduced.

Coronary heart disease (CHD)

The two main arteries that encircle the heart and supply it with blood are known as the coronary arteries. If you have diabetes, you have an increased risk of CHD, in which fatty deposits known as atheromas build up in your coronary arteries and restrict blood flow to your heart.

Causes

It is thought that a high level of insulin may be responsible for damage to the arteries (see High blood pressure). Other risk factors are high blood pressure, hyperlipidaemia, a high-fat diet, inactivity, smoking, obesity, a family history of CHD, and a blood glucose level that has been high for a period of years.

Symptoms and diagnosis

When the heart receives insufficient oxygen because blood flow through the coronary arteries is restricted, you may experience angina, a heart attack, or heart failure.

■ **ANGINA** A temporary sensation of pain or pressure in the chest is the main symptom of angina. You may also experience pain in your left

Q What is my risk of developing a circulatory condition?

A If you have diabetes and your blood glucose level is regularly above 7 millimoles per litre; your HbA1c test result is above 7 per cent; you smoke; you have high blood pressure (above 140/80 mmHg); a BMI above 30 (see p.46); or you are of South Asian, African, or Caribbean descent, you have a significant risk of developing a circulatory condition. Also, if you are a woman with diabetes, you lose extra protection against circulatory problems after menopause. If one or more of the above apply to you, you can still do a great deal to reduce your risk by making changes to your lifestyle, for example, by losing weight, being more physically active, or stopping smoking.

shoulder or down the inside of your left arm. This can happen when you are stressed or you exert yourself, for example, lifting a heavy object or walking faster than usual.

■ **HEART ATTACK** The main signs of a heart attack are severe chest pain, breathlessness, a pounding or irregular heartbeat, sweating, light-headedness, nausea, and sometimes loss of consciousness. Symptoms may also be few or mild.

■ **HEART FAILURE** The heart gradually loses its ability to pump blood around the body. Signs of heart failure include swelling in your legs, feet, and abdomen, fluid in your lungs, shortness of breath, and fatigue. The condition usually worsens slowly over time.

CHD may be diagnosed by an electrocardiogram (ECG) in which the heart's electrical impulses are

A temporary sensation of pain or pressure in the chest is the main symptom of angina. You may also experience pain in your left shoulder or down the inside of your left arm.

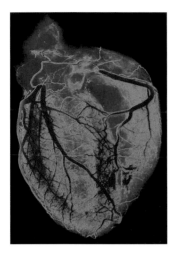

CORONARY ARTERIES
A network of arteries and veins supply blood to the heart so that it can be pumped around the body. Narrowing of the coronary arteries that supply the heart muscle can cause coronary heart disease.

The symptoms of a stroke depend on which part of the brain has been damaged. Your movement, speech, memory, vision, hearing, or balance may be affected.

recorded via electrodes placed on the skin. Imaging techniques using ultrasound waves and X-rays may be used to view the heart and assess the health of the coronary arteries.

Prevention and treatment

Lifestyle changes are the most important ways of preventing CHD: these include eating healthily, being physically active, stopping smoking, losing weight if necessary, reducing alcohol intake, and managing stress. Monitoring your blood pressure and blood lipid levels regularly and taking treatment if necessary will help. You can also help to prevent CHD by maintaining good long-term control of your diabetes. The treatment for CHD consists of tablets or surgery. Tablets include:

- Beta-blockers (see p.207).
- Nitrate-based drugs, such as isosorbide mononitrate and glyceryl trinitrate, which dilate the blood vessels around your heart.
- Anti-platelet drugs, such as aspirin, which prevent blood clotting.
- Calcium-channel blockers (see p.207).

The main surgical options for treating CHD are coronary artery bypass surgery and coronary angioplasty. Bypass surgery involves grafting a blood vessel from another part of your body and re-routing blood away from the damaged part of the artery. Coronary angioplasty involves feeding a fine tube into the blocked part of the artery and inflating a "balloon" at the end of the tube.

This widens the artery so that, when the balloon is deflated and removed, blood can flow unimpeded. A metal device known as a stent may also be implanted in an artery to keep it open.

If you have a heart attack and you are admitted to hospital, you will be treated with an insulin infusion followed by insulin injections at home for several months afterwards. This is to reduce your chances of having a further heart attack. You may or may not need to remain on insulin in the longer term, depending on your blood glucose control and other risk factors.

Outlook

There are very good prevention and treatment options for CHD, including tablets to reduce the risk of first or further heart attacks. However, a healthy lifestyle remains an extremely important part of keeping your circulation at its most efficient.

Stroke

When the blood flow to your brain is interrupted as a result of a blood clot or a burst blood vessel, your brain is deprived of oxygen and this causes some brain cells to die or be damaged.

Causes

The main risk factor for stroke is high blood pressure, which is a common complication in people with diabetes. Atherosclerosis (associated with high cholesterol in the blood), in which fatty deposits cause narrowing of the arteries, is another risk factor.

Symptoms and diagnosis

Stroke symptoms depend on which part of the brain has been damaged. Movement, speech, memory, vision, hearing, or balance may be affected. A stroke is diagnosed by your symptoms and/or a brain scan.

Prevention and treatment

If you have high blood pressure (see pp.206–208), keeping this well controlled by taking medication regularly and following guidelines for a healthy lifestyle can help to prevent stroke. Cutting down on saturated fat in food also helps to keep your circulation healthy. The treatment for stroke consists of assessment and rehabilitation of the functions affected; this may include physiotherapy and speech therapy.

Outlook

The outlook following a stroke depends on the functions that are affected – and how badly. Recovery may be possible with specialist help.

Peripheral vascular disease (PVD)

When fatty deposits build up in the arteries in the arms or legs, blood flow is restricted to the arm and leg muscles and this is known as peripheral vascular disease (PVD).

Causes

A high level of insulin circulating in the blood may be responsible for damage to the arteries (see High blood pressure). Other risk factors are high blood pressure, hyperlipidaemia, a high-fat diet, inactivity, smoking, obesity, and a blood glucose level that has been consistently high for a period of years.

Symptoms and diagnosis

The first sign of a narrowed arm or leg artery is pain and fatigue in the arm or calf muscles during physical activity caused by restricted blood flow (the greater the exertion, the greater the pain). PVD is diagnosed by your symptoms and history plus X-rays or ultrasound scans.

Prevention and treatment

The best way to prevent PVD is to combine healthy eating and physical activity with good long-term control of your diabetes. It can help to lose weight if you need to, stop smoking, and reduce your alcohol intake. It's important to have your blood pressure and blood lipid levels monitored and to take any treatment regularly. Treatment of PVD consists of anti-platelet drugs (see p.210), or calcium-channel blockers (see p.207). You may also be offered angioplasty or bypass surgery to replace the damaged artery (see p.210).

Outlook

The treatment for PVD either by medication or surgery can be very successful. However, reducing risk factors for further damage, especially by stopping smoking, will enhance their long-term success.

Practical tips

PREVENTING CARDIOVASCULAR CONDITIONS

- Eat healthily – including at least 5 portions of fruit and vegetables daily. Limit saturated fat.
- Do some physical activity, such as brisk walking for half an hour five times a week.
- Stop smoking.
- Keep your body mass index in the recommended range (see p.46).
- Keep your diabetes well controlled.
- Limit your alcohol consumption if you have been advised to do so.
- Make sure you take any medication you are prescribed to reduce your blood pressure or blood lipid levels.

Other conditions

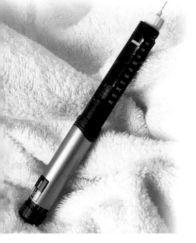

If you have had diabetes for a long time, you are susceptible to a number of conditions. Lumpy skin at insulin injection sites (lipohypertrophy) can develop if you repeatedly inject in the same site. Erectile dysfunction, also known as impotence, can occur as a result of nerve damage or blood flow problems, while damage to the nerves that control automatic bodily functions, such as your digestion and your body temperature is known as autonomic neuropathy.

Lipohypertrophy

Lumpy skin at insulin injection sites is known as lipohypertrophy. The lumps are swollen and raised, but not red or painful.

Causes

Repeated injections in the same injection site can cause fat deposits to accumulate under the skin. Insulin can also cause overgrowth of tissues where the skin is damaged. You are more likely to get lipohypertrophy if you use the same sites to inject your insulin for years, but it can develop after using the same site for only a few months.

Symptoms and diagnosis

Lumps usually develop slowly, so you may not notice that anything is wrong. Run your hand across your injection sites to assess whether the skin feels different there. If you can't feel any lumps but your blood glucose level fluctuates from day to day for no apparent reason, contact your health professional. Unpredictable swings in your blood glucose level indicate that you might be injecting into sites where cell growth is abnormal, which affects the absorption of your insulin. Your health professional will be able to tell you if you have lipohypertrophy by examining your injection sites.

Prevention and treatment

To avoid lipohypertrophy, don't inject into the same area each time (to find out where you can inject see p.97). If you already have lipohypertrophy, don't inject into any lumpy areas, even if injections there seem to feel less uncomfortable. If insulin absorption has been a problem, you may have increased your dose to combat this without knowing that lipohypertrophy was the problem. In this case, you may need to reduce your insulin dose by up to half when you use a new injection site to avoid hypos.

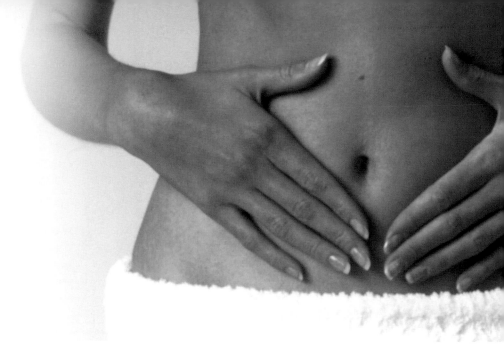

CHECKING INJECTION SITES
Repeatedly using the same injection site can cause lumpy skin, known as lipohypertrophy. Injecting into a different site each time will help prevent this. Check the skin at your injection sites regularly and, if you do feel any lumps, avoid injecting into that area.

Outlook

Over time, the lumps should reduce in size as fat cells are reabsorbed into your body. Large or long-standing lumps, however, may never disappear entirely, in which case you should never use these injection sites again.

Erectile dysfunction

Erectile dysfunction (ED), which is also known as impotence, is an inability to achieve or sustain an erection so that sexual intercourse can take place. The condition affects about one in three men who have diabetes and becomes more common with age.

Causes

Erectile dysfunction occurs as a result of a high blood glucose level over many years, which can damage your circulation and nerves, and lead to autonomic neuropathy (see p.215). As a result, the blood supply to the penis may be affected or nerve damage can affect the processes leading to sexual arousal. Erectile dysfunction may also be a side effect of drugs, including those used to lower blood pressure, for example beta blockers. There are other causes of ED that may or may not be related to your diabetes. These include depression, stress, anxiety, and relationship difficulties. Your risk of ED is also increased by heavy smoking and drinking. Rarely, ED is caused by low levels of testosterone or the hormone thyroxine. Discussing your symptoms and lifestyle with your health professional will help to identify which physical and/or psychological factors are involved in your ED.

Symptoms and diagnosis

Your ED is less likely to be diabetes-related if you have erections during the night or in the mornings, if your ED has developed suddenly, or if you

Erectile dysfunction affects about one in three men who have diabetes.

only suffer from ED in specific situations, such as when you feel stressed or when you are with a new partner. It is more likely to be linked to your diabetes if you are unable to achieve a erection at all and the problem has developed gradually. You may need tests to help identify the cause of ED, including a blood pressure check, physical examination, and a blood test to check testosterone and thyroxine levels. You may be tested for autonomic neuropathy (see right) or for peripheral neuropathy (see pp.200–202) because if other parts of your body are affected by nerve or circulation damage, diabetes may be a factor in your ED.

ED is more likely to be connected to your diabetes if you are unable to achieve a erection at all and the problem has developed gradually.

Prevention and treatment

The most important step you can take to prevent ED is to control your blood glucose. Initial treatment involves dealing with any underlying cause of your ED, for example if drug treatment is a likely cause, your health professional may suggest changing your medication. Low testosterone or thyroxine levels can also be treated with medication. Tight control of your blood glucose is very important and you may need to increase the dose of your tablets or insulin, or take a new medication to achieve this. You should also stop smoking and reduce your alcohol intake if you drink more than the safe amount (see p.38). If these measures do not restore your full sexual function, you may be offered further drug or physical treatments as well as counselling.

■ **DRUG TREATMENTS** The following drugs work by relaxing the muscles around the penis and improving blood flow to produce an erection.

● Alprostadil (Caverject) is inserted into the urethra in pellet form, or injected directly into the penis. Alprostadil can have side effects – your erection may not subside as normal after sexual activity and, if you use the injection form, bruising may occur around the injection site.

● Sildenafil (Viagra) or vardenafil (Levitra) are taken orally about one hour before sexual activity. Viagra can be effective for up to 6–8 hours; Levitra for up to 48 hours. They should not be taken with drugs containing nitrates, such as isosorbide mononitrate or glyceryl trinitrate, which you might be taking if you suffer from angina or high blood pressure, because the two together can cause very low blood pressure.

● Tadalafil (Cialis) is taken between 30 minutes and 12 hours before sexual activity. It works for up to 24 hours. It should not be taken with nitrates.

● Apomorphine hydrochloride (Uprima) is taken about 20 minutes before sexual activity. It is safe to take this drug with nitrates.

■ **PHYSICAL TREATMENTS** There are several physical aids that can help you to achieve and maintain an erection. The vacuum device consists of a plastic tube and rubber band that is placed over the penis. You use a pump to create a vacuum inside the tube, causing the penis to fill with blood and become erect. You then slip the rubber band onto the base of your penis to maintain your erection, and remove the tube and pump.

If blood vessels to your penis have become narrowed, surgery can restore normal blood flow. There is also a variety of penile implants available, from rods that keep the penis erect all the time (you fold your penis against your thigh or abdomen) to an inflatable device that is activated with a pump to hold the penis erect.

Outlook

Most treatments are effective and allow you to continue to enjoy lovemaking. However, they can make sex less spontaneous. Involving your partner in decisions about treating ED and incorporating that treatment into your lovemaking, can make your sex life more enjoyable. You may choose not to have treatment. ED does not adversely affect any other aspect of your diabetes nor your overall health.

Autonomic neuropathy

The nerves controlling parts of your body that you don't move voluntarily are the autonomic nerves. They help the body function by regulating your temperature, your heart rate, and your digestive system, for example. When these nerves are damaged, this is known as autonomic neuropathy.

Causes

Autonomic neuropathy is the result of consistently high blood glucose over many years. Damage to the nerves makes them less effective at transmitting impulses, which can affect your body's normal functions.

Symptoms and diagnosis

Autonomic neuropathy can produce a range of symptoms, including:
- Too much or too little sweating, very dry skin.
- Nausea, vomiting, diarrhoea or constipation.
- Dizziness (postural hypotension) when you stand up or get out of bed.
- Difficulty exercising because your heart rate does not increase/decrease.
- An inability to empty your bladder completely.
- Erectile dysfunction.
- Reduced awareness of hypos.

If you have more than one of the above symptoms, see your health professional to have your heart rate and blood pressure checked, as these are also under the control of your autonomic nervous system.

Prevention and treatment

Good blood glucose control helps to prevent autonomic neuropathy. Specific symptoms of the condition are treated as they occur. You may be prescribed medication to relieve nausea, vomiting, and diarrhoea, for example.

Outlook

Autonomic neuropathy is likely to be permanent, because the nerve damage cannot be repaired. Treatment is aimed at relieving your symptoms as they arise.

Practical tips

AVOIDING POSTURAL HYPOTENSION

- When you get up in the morning, sit on the edge of the bed for 5 minutes before standing up.

- Try keeping your head and shoulders raised while you sleep, perhaps on extra pillows or by adjusting your bed slightly, if you have an adjustable mattress.

- Ask your health professional whether wearing support stockings at night would help to relieve your symptoms.

Glossary

AUTONOMIC NEUROPATHY damage to the nerves that affect body functions such as digestion and body temperature.

BACKGROUND RETINOPATHY the first stage of retinopathy, in which blood vessels in the retina bulge and leak blood; some blood vessels have also closed down and have stopped supplying blood to the retina.

BETA CELLS cells in the pancreas that produce insulin.

BLOOD GLUCOSE LEVEL the concentration of glucose (sugar) in the blood, measured as the number of millimoles of glucose per litre of blood.

BMI (BODY MASS INDEX) height to weight ratio; the BMI is calculated by dividing body weight (in kilograms) by height (in metres) squared.

ERECTILE DYSFUNCTION inability to achieve or sustain an erection for sexual intercourse.

GESTATIONAL DIABETES diabetes developed during pregnancy that disappears after the baby is born.

GLUCAGON a hormone produced by the pancreas that raises the level of glucose in the blood by converting glycogen stored in the liver back into glucose.

GLUCOSE a simple sugar that is the body's primary energy source; most of the body's glucose supply comes from the digestion of carbohydrates and from glycogen stored in the liver being converted back into glucose.

GLYCOGEN the form in which glucose is stored in the liver.

GLYCOSYLATED HAEMOGLOBIN see HbA1c.

HBA1C (GLYCOSYLATED HAEMOGLOBIN) test that measures the level of glucose in the blood over the previous 6–8 weeks.

HYPERGLYCAEMIA a high blood glucose level – above 7 millimoles per litre.

HYPERLIPIDAEMIA high levels of fat in the blood.

HYPOGLYCAEMIA a low blood glucose level – below 4 millimoles per litre.

INFUSION fluid or insulin delivered continuously into a vein; infusions are usually carried out in hospital.

INJECTION SITE area of the body where insulin is injected.

INSULIN a pancreatic hormone produced to lower blood glucose by allowing glucose to enter body cells.

INSULIN DEVICE any device that is used to deliver insulin by injection.

INTERMEDIATE-ACTING INSULIN insulin that is injected once or twice daily, which has a peak of action between 4–8 hours after injection, providing a background supply of insulin.

ISCHAEMIA reduced blood supply to part of the body, due to narrowing of arteries.

KETOACIDOSIS a serious condition, caused by a very high blood glucose level, in which ketones are produced and the acid balance of the blood is affected.

KETONES acid by-products, produced from the breakdown of fat. Can be highly toxic if there is a severe lack of insulin.

LIPOHYPERTROPHY fatty lumps under the skin caused by repeatedly injecting into a small area of the body.

LIPOPROTEINS substances that consist of a protein combined with fat.

LONG-ACTING INSULIN insulin that is injected once a day and has a peak of action between 6–10 hours after injection, providing a background supply of insulin.

MICROALBUMINURIA very small amounts of protein in the urine; an early sign of nephropathy.

MILLIMOLES PER LITRE measure used to calculate blood glucose level.

MODY (MATURITY ONSET DIABETES OF THE YOUNG) diabetes with a specific genetic pattern, similar to Type 2 diabetes in its treatment.

NEPHRON the basic filtering unit of the kidney, consisting of a cluster of blood capillaries (glomerulus) and a long, thin tube (renal tubule); each kidney contains about one million nephrons.

NEPHROPATHY reduction in the kidneys' ability to function.

NEUROPATHY damage to the nerve supply in the body.

PANCREAS abdominal organ producing insulin, glucagon, and other digestive hormones.

PEAKLESS LONG-ACTING INSULIN a type of insulin that is injected once a day and that provides a background supply of insulin with no peak of action.

PERIPHERAL ISCHAEMIA reduced blood supply to legs and feet, due to narrowing of arteries.

PERIPHERAL NEUROPATHY damage to the nerves supplying the extremities of the body.

PREPROLIFERATIVE RETINOPATHY the second stage of retinopathy, in which new blood vessels start to form in the retina to replace those that have closed down; the new blood vessels are fragile and prone to bleeding.

PROLIFERATIVE RETINOPATHY the final stage of retinopathy, in which many new blood vessels form in the retina, often on top of existing blood vessels; the new blood vessels may bleed into the back of the eye, reducing vision.

PROTEINURIA large amounts of protein in the urine, a sign of permanent nephropathy.

RAPID-ACTING INSULIN a type of insulin injected at mealtimes that peaks within 1–2 hours after injection.

RETINAL DETACHMENT separation of the retina from its underlying layers; retinal detachment is a potential complication of retinopathy.

RETINOPATHY any disorder that affects the retina, usually due to damage to retinal blood vessels.

RUBEOTIC GLAUCOMA a potential complication of proliferative retinopathy in which the new blood vessels in the eye grow around the iris, which can cause visual impairment.

SHORT-ACTING INSULIN a type of insulin injected 20–40 minutes before mealtimes that peaks within 2–3 hours after injection.

TYPE 1 DIABETES diabetes in which the beta cells in the pancreas have been destroyed and, as a result, the body can no longer produce insulin.

TYPE 2 DIABETES diabetes in which the body cells are resistant to the action of insulin and insulin production gradually declines.

VITREOUS HAEMORRHAGE bleeding into the rear of the eye, a temporary condition that is a potential complication of retinopathy.

Useful addresses

The following organizations provide useful information; some also offer support or can help you to make contact with other people who have diabetes. You can also obtain details about further sources of information from your health professional.

British Association for Counselling and Psychotherapy
BACP House
15 St John's Business Park
Lutterworth LE17 4HB
Tel: 01455 883300
Website: *www.bacp.co.uk*

Diabetes Research and Wellness Foundation
101–102 Northney Marina
Hayling Island PO11 0NH
Tel: 023 9263 7808
Website: *www.drwf.org.uk*

Diabetes UK
10 Parkway
London NW1 7AA
General enquires: 020 7424 1000
Careline: 0845 120 2960, or email on careline@diabetes.org.uk
Website: *www.diabetes.org.uk*

Disability Alliance
Universal House
88–94 Wentworth Street
London E1 7SA
Tel: 020 7247 8776
Helpline: 020 7247 8763
Website: *www.disabilityalliance.org*

Driver and Vehicle Licensing Agency (DVLA)
DVLA Swansea
SA6 7JL
Tel: 0870 600 0301
Website: *www.dvla.gov.uk*

Diabetes Trust
PO Box 294
Northampton NN1 4XS
Tel: 01604 622837
Website: *www.iddtinternational.org*

Juvenile Diabetes Research Foundation
19 Angel Gate
City Road
London EC1V 2PT
Tel: 020 7713 2030
Website: *www.jdrf.org.uk*

Medic-Alert Foundation
1 Bridge Wharf,
156 Caledonian Road,
London N1 9UU
Tel: 020 7833 3034
Helpline: 0800 581 420
Website: *www.medicalert.org.uk*

National Kidney Federation
The Point
Coach Road
Shireoaks
Worksop S81 8BW
Tel: 01909 487 795
Website: *www.kidney.org.uk*

Royal National Institute for Blind People
105 Judd Street
London WC1H 9NE
Tel: 020 7388 1266
Website: *www.rnib.org.uk*

Sexual Dysfunction Association
Suite 301 Emblem House
London Bridge Hospital
27 Tooley Street
London SE1 2PR
Helpline: 0870 7743 571
Website: *www.sda.uk.net*

Stroke Association
Stroke House,
240 City Road
London EC1V 2PR
Tel: 020 7566 0300
Helpline: 0845 303 3100
Website: *www.stroke.org.uk*

Successful Diabetes
PO Box 819
Northampton NN4 4AG
Tel: 08445 617205
Website: *www.successfuldiabetes.com*

To contact other people with diabetes, try the following sites:
www.diabetes-insight.info
www.insulin-pumpers.org.uk

For specific information, try:
www.diabetes-exercise.org
www.glycaemicindex.com

Another useful source is the American Diabetes Association
Website: *www.diabetes.org*

Index

A

abscesses, foot ulcers 205
acarbose 80–81, 102
ACE inhibitors 139, 199, 207
acne 177
acromegaly 17, 112
adrenaline 104, 131, 177, 179, 207
air travel 123
alcohol 38, 39–40, 66, 103–4, 179–80
alprostadil 214
amniotic fluid 142
amputation, feet 203, 205
analogue insulin 84–5
angina 209, 214
angioplasty 203, 210, 211
animal insulin 84
annual reviews 21, 26, 150–1
antenatal care 139, 140, 144
antibiotics 176, 205
anticonvulsants 202
antidepressants 189, 202
anti-platelet drugs 210, 211
arteries
    coronary heart disease 209
    high blood pressure 206
    peripheral ischaemia 202–5
    peripheral vascular disease 211
athlete's foot 129
autonomic neuropathy 215

B

babies
    birth 143
    looking after new baby 146–7
    problems during pregnancy 141, 142
    Type 1 diabetes 154
bacteria 131
basal-bolus regimen 90
beta-blockers 17, 133, 207, 210, 213
birth 141, 142–3, 145
bladder problems 19, 137
blisters, feet 129
blood glucose 10–15
    children 157–61, 162 167–9
    controlling 23–4, 76–81, 83
    diet and 30–3
    exercise and 56–9
    hyperglycaemia 23, 25, 110–13
    hypoglycaemia 23, 24–5, 102–9
    illness and 131–2
    long-term drug treatments and 133–4
    menstrual cycle and 136–7, 177
    monitoring 22–3, 62–75
    pre-conception 138
    in pregnancy 140, 144–5
    safe levels 22, 65
    sex and 126–7
    while in hospital 134–5
blood glucose tests
    children 159, 167–8
    diagnosing diabetes 20, 21
    equipment 67–70
    frequency 64
    high readings 74–5
    low readings 75
    meters 67, 68–71
    performing 70–1
    in pregnancy 139
blood pressure 21
    postural hypotension 215
    see also high blood pressure
blood vessels
    cardiovascular conditions 206–11
    foot problems 128
    kidney problems 197
    peripheral ischaemia 202–5
    peripheral vascular disease 211
    retinopathy 190–4
blurred vision 19, 195
body mass index 21, 45–6
body shape 16, 45
bone problems 204, 205
bowel problems 134
brain, stroke 210–11
breastfeeding 144, 145, 146–7, 156
burns, feet 130

C

Caesarean section 141, 142, 145
calcium-channel blockers 207, 210, 211
calories 49–51, 53, 54
cancer 134
Candida albicans 137
cannabis 180–1
capsaicin creams 202

carbohydrates 33–6
 carbohydrate counting 35–6
 children and 156
 controlling diabetes 24, 30–1
 digestion 10–11
 glycaemic index (GI) 34–5
 for hypoglycaemia 107
cardiovascular conditions 27,
  206–11
cartridges, insulin 95–6
cataracts 27, 194–5
Charcot foot 205
children 12, 15, 154–69
 blood glucose control 157–61,
  162, 167–9
 food 156–7
 hypoglycaemia 158, 159–61,
  164, 168–9
 school-age children 162–9
cholesterol 202, 208
coma 19, 113, 132
complications, long-term 26–7,
  65
conception 138–9
contraception 126–7, 138, 181
corns 129–30
coronary heart disease 209–10
cortisol 104, 131, 177, 179
counselling, for depression 189
Cushing's disease 17, 112
cystic fibrosis 17
cystitis 19, 137

D

dehydration 12, 18, 131,
  132–3, 181
depression 27, 52, 147, 175,
  186–9
diabetes
 causes 16–17
 diagnosis 20–1

long-term complications
  26–7, 65
 looking after yourself 22–7
 symptoms 12, 18–19
 types of 12–16
 see also Type 1 diabetes;
  Type 2 diabetes
diabetic ketoacidosis 113, 131,
  132, 161
diabetic products 38
diagnosis 20–1
dialysis, kidney 198, 199
diaries, monitoring blood glucose
  73, 74, 91
diarrhoea 131, 132–3
diet see food
digestive system 10–11
disabled, registering as 119
diuretics 17, 133, 207
Down's syndrome 16
DPP4 inhibitors 81
drinks 38–40
driving 120–2, 176, 177, 195
drugs
 and causes of diabetes 17
 drug interactions 79
 free prescriptions 182
 and hypoglycaemia 24
 long-term treatments 133–4
 over-the-counter 133
 recreational drugs 180–1
 see also tablets

E

eating out 41–3, 93–4, 157,
  166
electrocardiography 207, 209–10
end-stage renal failure 196,
  198, 199
equipment
 insulin injections 95–100

monitoring 67–73
 when travelling 122–4
erectile dysfunction 127, 213–15
exercise see physical activity
eye conditions 19, 21, 27,
  190–5
 cataracts 194–5
 during pregnancy 142
 retinopathy 138, 139, 190–4

F

fasting 32, 94–5
fasting blood glucose test 20, 21
fat, subcutaneous 98
fats, in diet 36–7, 51, 208–9
fevers 131, 132
fibrates 208
fingerprick test 20, 21
fits 160
fluid retention 197, 198
fluorescein angiography 192–3
food
 and children 156–7, 164–6
 controlling diabetes 24,
  30–3
 cooking 40–1
 eating out 41–3
 groups 33–40
 and hyperglycaemia 111
 labels 50
 poisoning 125, 131
 and teenagers 176
foot conditions 27, 200–5
footcare 21, 59, 125, 128–30, 202

G

gangrene 203, 205
genetics 16, 17
gestational diabetes 12,
  16–17, 83, 121, 144–5
glaucoma 192, 193, 194

glibenclamide 79
gliclazide 79
glimepiride 79
GLP1 analogues 81
glucagon 10–11, 102, 107–8, 109
glucose
    for hypoglycaemia 102, 106, 108
glycaemic index 34–5
glycogen 10, 56, 83
growth hormone 157, 162, 174, 177

H

haemochromatosis 17
haemodialysis 198, 199
HbA1c test 23, 62–3, 66, 67, 77, 139, 176
health checks 148–51
heart attack 209, 210
heart disease 57, 209–10
heart monitoring 207, 209–10
heat, and hypoglycaemia 104–5, 125
high blood pressure 21, 37, 206–8
    causes 206
    diagnosis 206–7
    drug treatment 133, 139, 207
    and kidney damage 198–9
    prevention 207
    and retinopathy 191
    and stroke 210
holidays 66, 122–5
hormones
    disorders 17
    hormone replacement therapy (HRT) 137
    and hyperglycaemia 111–12, 131

menstrual cycle 136–7, 177
stress hormones 131, 179
teenage 177
hospitals 134–5
hyperglycaemia 23, 25, 110–13
    causes and prevention 110–12
    illness and 131
    risks 113
    symptoms 112
    treatment 112–13
hyperlipidaemia 208–9
hypoglycaemia 23, 24–5, 102–9
    alcohol and 39–40, 179–80
    causes and prevention 102–5
    in children 158, 159–61, 164, 168–9
    illness and 132
    new babies and 146–7
    in pregnancy 140
    recovery period 108–9
    sex and 126–7
    symptoms 105–6
    in teenagers 178
    treatment 106–8
    while driving 120–2, 176
hypotension, postural 215

I

illness 130–5
    adjusting insulin doses 94
    children and 161
    and hyperglycaemia 111
    long-term drug treatments 133–4
    monitoring blood glucose 66
    over-the-counter medicines 133
    teenagers 179

immune system 15, 17, 101
immunosuppressant drugs 17
impotence 213–15
injections 24, 76, 77, 82, 94
    children 159, 167–8
    and hypoglycaemia 103
    injection devices 95–7, 98
    injection sites 97
    skin problems 212–13
    techniques 98–9
    teenagers 174–5, 177
insulin 10–12
    adjusting doses 90–5
    blood glucose control 66, 83
    checking appearance of 98
    children 157, 159–61, 164
    controlling diabetes with 31–3, 35–6, 82–101
    eating out 41–2, 93–4
    gestational diabetes 144
    hyperglycaemia 112, 113
    hypoglycaemia 102–9
    and illness 131, 132
    inhaled insulin 100, 101
    insulin resistance 15, 206, 208
    physical activity and 56–9
    in pregnancy 138–40, 145
    pumps 90, 96–7
    regimens 87–90
    side effects 87
    storage 99, 124
    strength and doses 83–4
    teenagers 174–5, 177–8
    Type 1 diabetes 12–15
    Type 2 diabetes 14, 15
    types of 84–7
    and weight gain 46–7
    when travelling 122–4
    while in hospital 135

insurance 121, 122
intermediate-acting insulin 86–7
ischaemia, peripheral 202–5
islets of Langerhans 10, 12, 100–1

J

jet-injectors, needle-free 96
joint problems 134

K

ketoacidosis 19, 113
ketones 19, 51, 113, 132, 140, 141
kidney conditions 27, 196–9

L

labour 141, 142–3, 145
lancets 67–8
lancing devices 67–8, 72
laser treatment 194
lipohypertrophy 212–13
long-term complications 26–7, 65
lung disease 134

M

macrosomia 142
maculopathy 193, 194
Maturity Onset Diabetes of the Young (MODY) 12, 16, 76, 82–3, 170
medicines *see* drugs; tablets
menopause 112, 137
menstrual cycle 112, 136–7, 177
meters, blood glucose 67, 68–71
metformin 78–9, 80–1, 102, 199
microalbuminuria 196, 197, 199
minerals 37
monitoring diaries 73, 74, 91
morning sickness 140

N

nateglinide 80
needle-clipping devices 100
needle-free jet-injectors 96
needles
    disposal of 100
    insulin injections 95–6
    lancets 67–8
    phobias 95
nephropathy 196–9
nervous system
    autonomic neuropathy 215
    foot problems 128
    peripheral neuropathy 200–2
nitrates 210, 214
non-ketotic hyperosmolar state 113, 132

O

oestrogen 136, 177
ophthalmoscopy 192
oral glucose tolerance test 20, 21
osteomyelitis 204
over-the-counter medicines 133

PQ

packed lunches 165–6
pancreas 10, 12, 17, 101
pancreatitis 17
peakless long-acting insulin 86, 87
penis, erectile dysfunction 127, 213–15
peripheral ischaemia 201, 202–5
peripheral neuropathy 200–2, 203, 204–5
peripheral vascular disease 211
peritoneal dialysis 198, 199
physical activity 52–9
    adjusting insulin doses 94

controlling diabetes 24
dieting and 50–1
and hyperglycaemia 111
and hypoglycaemia 104
monitoring blood glucose 65
teenagers 178
pioglitazone 79, 80
polyhydramnios 142
postural hypotension 215
pre-eclampsia 142
pregnancy 126, 127, 138–47, 181
    gestational diabetes 12, 16–17, 83, 121, 144–5
    monitoring blood glucose 65
    planning 138–9
    and retinopathy 191–2
progesterone 136
proteins 36
proteinuria 196, 197–8, 199
pumps, insulin 90, 96–7

R

random blood glucose test 20, 21
rapid-acting insulin 84–5, 86
rebound hypoglycaemia 109
relationships 126–7, 181
renal disease 196–9
repaglinide 80
retina 21, 27
retinal detachment 193, 194
retinopathy 138, 139, 190–4
rosiglitazone 79, 80
rubeotic glaucoma 193, 194

S

salt 37, 199
saxagliptin 81
school-age children 162–9
school meals 165–6
school trips 166–7

sex 126–7, 181, 213–15
shift work 120
shoes 128, 130, 205
short-acting insulin 85–6
sight problems 19, 192–5
Sitagliptin 81
skin
    injection sites 97, 212–13
    teenage problems 176, 177
sleep, and hypoglycaemia 147
smoking 180, 202, 207
snacks 33, 57, 58–9
    children and 156, 157, 160, 164–5
soluble insulin 85–6
sport 178
statins 208
steroids 17, 134
stomach upsets 125, 131
storing insulin 99, 124
stress
    and hyperglycaemia 111–12, 131
    and hypoglycaemia 104, 147
    teenagers and 175
stress hormones 131, 179
stroke 210–11
sugar 33–4, 38
sulphonylureas 59, 79, 102
sweeteners 38
symptoms 12, 18–19
    in children 154, 162
    hyperglycaemia 25
    hypoglycaemia 24–5, 105–6
    in teenagers 170, 177
syringes 96, 99, 100

T
tablets
    and breastfeeding 144
    controlling diabetes 24, 76–81
    and hyperglycaemia 112
    and illness 131
    and kidney problems 199
    and physical activity 59
    and pregnancy 138, 145
    reminders 79
teenagers 170–83
testing strips 67, 68, 70–1, 72
testosterone 177, 213, 214
tests
    diagnosing diabetes 20–1
    eye tests 192
    see also blood glucose tests; urine tests
thiazide diuretics 17, 133
thiazolidinediones 79–80, 102
thirst 12, 18
thrush 19, 137
tiredness 18–19
toenails, cutting 128–9, 130
transplants 100–1, 199
travel 122–5, 166–7
Type 1 diabetes 12–15
    in children 154, 162
    diagnosis 21
    illness and 132
    insulin injections 76, 82, 86–7, 89, 90
    symptoms 18
    teenagers 170
    weight and 44
Type 2 diabetes 12, 15
    after gestational diabetes 145
    in children 162
    controlling 24
    diagnosis 21
    illness and 132–3
    insulin injections 77, 82–3, 87, 89
    symptoms 18
    tablets 76–7
    teenagers 170
    weight and 44–5

U
ulcers, foot 128, 201, 203, 204–5
ultrasound scans 139, 198
unconsciousness 106, 107–8, 109, 160
urine
    increased urination 12, 18
    kidney conditions 196–9
urine tests 20, 21
    for kidney problems 197–8
    monitoring blood glucose 63
    in pregnancy 139, 144

V
vaginal problems 19, 127, 137
vasodilators 17
vegetarian diet 32
verrucae 129
Vildagliptin 81
viruses 17, 131
vision problems 19, 192–5
vitreous haemorrhage 193, 194
vomiting 132–3, 140, 161

WXYZ
waist size 45
warning signs, hypoglycaemia 105, 106
weight control 44–51
    risk factors for diabetes 15, 16
    teenagers 170, 174–5
weight loss, symptom of diabetes 12, 19, 44, 46
women's health 136–47
work 118–20

Acknowledgments

Authors' acknowledgments We would like to thank the following people for their support and contributions: Stuart Bootle; Jane, Jake, and Charlie Buckingham; Shelley Foster; Iain, Vicky, Daniel, and Emma Levitt; Steven Sexton; Joe Solowiejczyk; Nick Steiner; Janet Sumner; Sophie Thomas; Graham Toms; George Walker; Jan Williamson; and the staff of The Hollies medical centre. We would also like to thank the many others who have contributed along the way, providing information and support at crucial times while we were writing. In addition, the editorial and design teams of Dorling Kindersley and Cooling Brown have been invaluable in helping us to understand the world of publishing. We have also received strong support and endless encouragement from our friends, families, and close colleagues. We hope all of you will celebrate and enjoy the final product.

Photographer Trish Gant

Models Charlie Buckingham, Jake Buckingham, Jane Buckingham, Angela Cameron, Sagaren Pillay, Nicholas Steiner, George Walker, Jeremy Wallis, Jan Williamson.

Index Hilary Bird

Picture credits

Alamy: Mark Harmel 6bl; Epictura 136tl; Image100 148tl; Jack Sparticus 157br; Image Source 163tr; Mark Harmel 177br. **Corbis**: John Henley 2; John Henley 19tr; Roy Botterell 30tl; Roy Botterell 31tr; Ronnie Kaufman 47br; Thom Lang 76tl; Jose Luis Pelaez, Inc. 77tr; © LWA – Dann Tardif 103tr; Steve Prezant 111tr; Ford Smith 126bl; Ken Redding 129tr; Mark M Lawrence 137tr; Charles Gupton 165br; 171tr; Kevin Fleming 178b; © LWA – Dann Tardif 184; 206tl. **Dorling Kindersley**: David Murray and Jules Selmes 42bcl; David Murray and Jules Selmes 42br; Simon Brown 154tl; Simon Brown 155tr. **Getty**: Taxi/Stephen Derr 7bc; Image Bank/Romilly Lockyer 8; Taxi/Gary Buss 10tl; Photographer's Choice/Nancy Brown 16bl; Taxi/Gary Buss 23tr; Photodisc Red 26bl; Taxi/Dan Kenyon 28; Photographer's Choice/Robin Macdougall 33br; Image Bank/Garry Gay 36bla; Image Bank/Rita Maas 36bl; Taxi/Antonio Mo 43cra; Stone/Steven Peters 45tr; Image Bank/Sean Justice 52tl; Taxi/Stephen Derr 53tr; Stone/David Madison 55br; Image Bank/Yellow Dog Productions 59b; Taxi/Justin Pumfrey 60; Taxi/Arthur Tilly 66bl; Thinkstock 74b; Image Bank/Marc Romanelli 81br; Image Bank/Daly & Newton 114; Taxi/Peter Denton 116tl; Taxi/Michael Goldman 117tr; Image Bank/Color Day Production 119br; Stone/Klaus Lahnstein 123b; Image Bank/Peter Mason 124bl; Photodisc Green 128tl; Taxi/Michael Goldman 133br; Image Bank/Tracy Frankel 141b; Photographer's Choice/Jim Bastardo 143br; Stone/Roger Charity 146bl; Thinkstock 149tr; Taxi/Antonio Mo 152; Taxi/Jim Franco 162tl; Foodpix/Burke/Triolo Productions 166b; Stone/Steve Taylor 170tl; Taxi/David Oliver 183br; Taxi/Jim Cummins 186tl; Taxi/Bill Ling 187tr; Stone/Dave Crosier 190tl; Taxi/Arthur Tilly 191tr; Image Bank/Thierry Dosogne 196tl; Stone/Elie Bernager 197tr; Stone/David Joel 207tr; Photodisc Green 172b. **SPL**: Gusto 11tr; CNRI 12bc; Astrid & Hanns-Frieder Michler 12br; BSIP, Chassenet 18tl; Faye Norman 20tl; Ruth Jenkinson/MIDIRS 20bl; Geoff Tompkinson 192bl; Custom Medical Stock Photo 193cr; Paul Parker 193br; Sue Ford 195bl; Mauro Fermariello 199br; Josh Sher 204tl; 210tl; Saturn Stills 212tl; BSIP Barrelle 213tr

All other images © Dorling Kindersley.
For further information see **www.dkimages.com**

Rosemary Walker, RGN, BSc (Hons), FETC worked as a diabetes specialist nurse for 16 years. She is a former chair of the Royal College of Nursing's Diabetes Nursing Forum and was a member of the UK Government's Expert Reference Group, which set national standards in diabetes care.

Formerly a nurse specializing in diabetes, **Jill Rodgers, RGN, MSc, BA (Hons)** later established the National Diabetes Facilitators Group, which she chaired for six years, and played a key role in the foundation of the Journal of Diabetes Nursing. Since 1996, she has been working with an international team on "Learning for Life" programmes promoting empowerment for people with diabetes.

Together, Rosemary and Jill are partners in Successful Diabetes and provide help and support for people living with diabetes, via their website www.successfuldiabetes.com and through the workshops they run.